MediScams

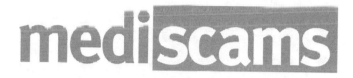

mediscams

How to Spot and Avoid
Health Care Scams,
Medical Frauds, and
Quackery from the Local
Physician to the Major
Health Care Providers and
Drug Manufacturers

Chuck Whitlock

foreword by Ben Chandler, Attorney General, Kentucky

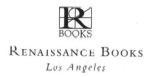

RENAISSANCE BOOKS
Los Angeles

ISBN: 1-58063-180-0

10 9 8 7 6 5 4 3 2 1

Design by Lisa-Theresa Lenthall

Published by Renaissance Books
Distributed by St. Martin's Press
Manufactured in the United States of America
First edition

Important Note

I encourage you to actively participate in improving your own health care. You must be responsible for determining what's appropriate for your needs. The information, data, and statements contained in *MediScams* are not intended nor implied to be a substitute for professional medical advice. Always seek the advice and opinions of your physician or other qualified health care provider prior to starting any new treatment or with any questions you may have regarding your condition.

Nothing contained in *MediScams* is intended for diagnosis or treatment. The material in *MediScams* is general in nature and is intended for informational use only. The information contained herein is not meant to imply endorsement or recommendation. It is not intended, and must not be taken, to be the provision or practice of medical, nursing, or professional health care advice or services in any jurisdiction. It does not cover all possible uses, actions, precautions, side effects, or interactions of any medical treatments, nor is the information intended as medical advice for individual problems or for making an evaluation as to the risks and benefits of taking a particular drug, supplement, treatment, or other medical-related service.

In no event will the Publisher, Author, Editors, or Distributors of this book be held liable for any decision made or action taken by you or anyone else in reliance upon the information provided in *MediScams*. In no event shall the Publisher, Author, Editors, or Distributors be liable for any direct, indirect, incidental, consequential, special, exemplary, punitive or any other monetary or other damages, fees, fines, penalties, or liabilities arising out of or relating in any way to the information provided in *MediScams*.

The stories you're about to read are real. However, some victims' names, dates, and specific locations were changed to disguise the identity of some of those involved. In some cases, this was done to protect the anonymity of victims who are embarrassed or fearful of retribution since they stepped forward to report the crime or testify against their perpetrators. In other cases, the perpetrator has not been tried in a court of law yet, or a known con artist is still wanted, and I don't want to jeopardize the case. If a victim has committed suicide, there is no reason to cause the family additional grief or notoriety. None of the changes materially affects the stories or lessons to be learned.

To the physicians, surgeons, nurses, and other trained,
professional medical practitioners who are dedicated and perform
their services to the highest possible standards,
in spite of the tremendous pressures to do otherwise.

Contents

Acknowledgments

A book about health care is a daunting undertaking. Just sifting through the volumes of medical records, police files, and scientific data could take a lifetime. Thanks to the following people, the job of writing this book was made manageable. Due in large measure to their respective contributions, I hope *MediScams* will address the health care concerns and interests of people seeking medical care for years to come.

Special thanks to my brother, Bill Whitlock, for being there when our Ma went through her medical ordeal and for reliving the experience in such great detail for me.

This book wouldn't have been possible without Jim Schutte, Ph.D., Gail Wayper, and Candace Whitlock. Many thanks to my manager and friend, Peter Miller, and to Richard O'Connor, my publishing editor.

My ongoing thanks to Oprah Winfrey and David Boul, who launched my television and true-crime writing careers.

My heartfelt appreciation to the following for their contributions: San Diego Deputy District Attorney Stacy Running; Stephen Barrett, M.D.; Attorney General Ben Chandler of the great state of Kentucky; Kentucky's Consumer Protection Division Director, Todd Leatherman; Ken Hunter, President of the Council of Better Business Bureaus; U.S.P.S. Inspector Bob Kuykendall; Homicide Detective Chris Peterson (Retired);

producer extraordinaire John Stevens; John Dodes, D.D.S.; Bob McCoy; Vincent Bugliosi; Ben Wilson, M.D.; William Jarvis, Ph.D.; Sharene Rekow; Gerry Wilson; Tracy McLarney; Neil Kingery; C. J. Pederson; Phil Van Auken; Peter Unsinger, Ph.D.; Richard Brinkley; Maureen O'Boyle; Ann Rule; Lavoyed Hudgins; John Hess, M.D.; Gene Koppenhaver; Lee Rooklin; Greg Branson; Russ Gorsline; Steve Anderson; Trace Skeen; Daniel Highkin, M.D.; Frank Abagnale; FBI agents Alan J. Peters and Joanne Yakshe; Ted Doyle; David Kessler, C.F.E.; Faye O'Bryant; and Dan Mihalko, Chris Correal, and Marie Timms of the U.S. Postal Service. Thanks also to Alan James, Eric Epperson, Barbara Forster, and Nanci James.

This is only a partial list of all who responded to my plea for assistance. The list includes physicians, surgeons, police officers, prosecutors, friends in the media, and folks afflicted with almost every imaginable malady. Some suffer with terminal conditions; a few have gone into remission. Many have died.

I must also acknowledge the pain and suffering of the nameless, faceless victims of medical quackery. We share this collective work as part of our legacy.

Foreword

As the attorney general for the state of Kentucky, it's my sworn duty to prosecute crimes committed by people and companies who defraud and abuse our citizens. Being defrauded by a telemarketer or an investment scammer can rob a person of their money and trust, but being defrauded in the medical arena also can rob a person of their health or life.

When Chuck asked me to write a foreword for this book, I was very pleased. His continuous efforts to help consumers learn the tricks of the con artists are to be commended. Chuck's journalistic investigations into white collar crime are well known, as are his award-winning television reports on programs such as *Extra, Hard Copy,* and *Inside Edition.* He has shared his investigations and stories with hundreds of Kentucky consumers and law-enforcement professionals attending "Scam Jams" which my office sponsored, helping us to earn an award from the National Association of Consumer Agency Administrators.

Among the most chilling of Chuck's investigations are those involving patient abuse and Medicaid and Medicare fraud. His investigation exposing the failure of nursing homes to conduct state-required background checks—resulting in their hiring Chuck, who was using the identity of a felon—is truly disturbing. In addition, he has posed as a nursing-home administrator, recording Medicare providers offering substantial kickbacks and suggesting he allow unnecessary medical tests and treatments in order to make more money.

It is critical that we all learn as much as we can to protect ourselves. Education and public awareness are the keys to keeping you and your loved ones safe.

The Honorable Albert B. Chandler III
Attorney General, State of Kentucky

(The Office of the Kentucky Attorney General consulted with the Kentucky Executive Branch Ethics Branch prior to publication of this Foreword. The Office of the Kentucky Attorney General does not receive and is not responsible for the disposition of any funds paid for the purchase of this book.)

Introduction

What is a "MediScam"? Quite simply, it is any practice that takes in health care dollars under false pretenses. That broad definition certainly encompasses deliberate frauds, such as unlicensed doctors who perform surgery, sellers of bogus or counterfeit "medicines" that are of no conceivable benefit, and those who bill Medicare or other health insurance for services that were either unnecessary or were never provided in the first place. Those are the easy ones to identify. Unfortunately, they're not the only MediScams out there.

MediScams also include products and services that may be offered honestly and with the best of intentions, but are of no clinical benefit. Take the case of "Therapeutic Touch" —the concept that the practitioner (usually a nurse) can "realign the body's energy field" by moving his or her hands along the patient's body without actually touching it. Although this "therapy" was developed by otherwise competent and highly respected nursing professionals, neither the proponents nor the practitioners of Therapeutic Touch are able to demonstrate that human "energy fields" even exist, let alone that they can be manipulated by another person. All it took was a science fair project by a curious nine-year-old girl to thoroughly debunk this nonexistent "therapy."

Likewise, there are proponents of every manner of dietary supplement, from vitamin C to shark cartilage, who honestly believe there's a supplement to prevent or cure every known disease—they just can't prove it. These people may not be frauds, in that they are not deliberately deceiving their customers; still, they are MediScammers in the sense that, like the snake-oil salesmen of yore, they make unproven and unjustified claims about the products and services they are selling—and profit by doing so.

Even major pharmaceutical manufacturers have been known to deceive consumers for profit. Take the case of the weight loss drug combination popularly known as "phen-fen." Although it was touted as a safe way to lose weight, in this book I'll show you why the drugs' manufacturer had adequate reason to know all along that the two drugs that make up phen-fen were potentially lethal when prescribed together.

Sometimes the mainstream medical community itself participates, however unwittingly, in MediScams. Take, for example, the well-intentioned doctors who prescribed phen-fen, not knowing that they were sending some of their patients into cardiac surgery—or the grave.

The cost of MediScams is staggering. In financial terms, it has been estimated that simple fraud accounts for as much as 10 percent of total annual health care expenditures of $1 trillion, a figure that includes the cheating of government programs such as Medicare. *Health care fraud is costing us over $100 billion a year, folks! That works out to $4,000 per person!* And the result is increased health insurance premiums and Medicare taxes for all of us.

Partially because of fraudulent losses to MediScams, medical insurance is becoming unaffordable for many Americans. According to the U.S. census, 44.3 million Americans remain uninsured. Who knows how many are *under*insured? Here's the double-edged sword: By helping to make legitimate health care unaffordable, MediScams drive more and more of us to seek less expensive alternatives—which are often other MediScams. And so goes the vicious cycle.

It is tragic that the nation which turns out perhaps the world's best-trained medical practitioners—not to mention the technology that enables surgeons to transplant nearly every organ except the brain—can leave so many of its own citizens uninsured and without access to lifesaving care. In the event of their greatest crisis, many Americans are left abandoned with nowhere to turn.

Even having medical insurance and a good doctor is no guarantee that you won't be victimized. Many patients have paid health insurance premiums for decades without filing a single claim. Yet when they are diagnosed with a serious condition, their insurance carrier denies payment for treatment because their doctor wants to pursue a treatment that the carrier deems "experimental." Organ transplants and cutting-edge cancer treatments are commonly denied on this basis. Never mind that other insurance companies may be paying for the same procedures—and possibly enjoying a high cure rate. The more expensive your prescribed treatment, the more likely it is to be denied.

Many of the problems I discuss in the chapter on health maintenance organizations (HMOs) are not unique to HMOs or other managed-care plans. All types of health insurance companies have dissatisfied customers. I chose to focus on HMOs for three reasons: First, 85 percent of all Americans who have health insurance are enrolled in an HMO or other managed-care plan. Second, most HMOs and related plans are practically immune from civil liability thanks to the Employee Retirement Income Security Act of 1974 (ERISA). That means that if your HMO qualifies under ERISA, it can refuse to provide you with even lifesaving medical care without worrying that you might sue. Third, I selected HMOs because those in managed-care plans tend to be less confident about America's health care system than those in fee-for-services plans; and those in HMOs are less satisfied than those in other types of managed-care plans according to a recent Health Confidence Survey.

What would the quality of your life be if other profit-making companies didn't have to worry about civil litigation? What if your home was damaged by fire and your insurance company refused to pay a dime because repairing your house was considered "experimental" or unnecessary? What if your new car broke down and had to sit in the shop for six months while awaiting approval of the needed repairs under warranty? You could sue those companies for damages. Yet when your health or even your life is at stake, an HMO can refuse you treatment on the grounds that it is experimental or unnecessary, or they can drag their feet for months before authorizing it. And there's little you can do about it.

In the HMO's or other health insurer's ideal scenario, you pay premiums your entire life, never get sick, then drop dead of a heart attack and are transported directly to the funeral home. That's the reality of business, and there's nothing wrong with it as long as good health care is there for you if and when you need it. HMOs become MediScammers, however, when you complain of chest pains to your primary-care physician, yet that doctor—because it will cost him or her money—refuses to refer you to a cardiologist or to order the tests that might determine whether you are, in fact, suffering heart problems. It happens all the time, and patients die as a result.

Another problem for health care consumers is their rising expectations. Medical miracles have become commonplace. The blind are made to see, the paralyzed are given back the use of their bodies, an incurable disease is cured. Desperate patients reason that surely there's a cure out there for inoperable cancers and multiple sclerosis (MS) and every other known disease. And whenever authentic medicine doesn't have the answers based on scientific evidence, it creates a void that the MediScammers rush to fill.

"Yes," says the MediScammer, "there is a cure, and I have it. Furthermore, I'm the only one who can offer it to you because the rest of the medical community is suppressing my research." And the patient who falls for this line loses not only money but the time that could have been far better spent seeking legitimate health care.

This book is intended to present a broad overview of MediScams to show how pervasive they are and to reveal the common patterns of how they work. I'm not attempting to present an in-depth, encyclopedic review of the subject because, quite simply, there are many more MediScams out there than could possibly be covered adequately in one book.

Notably missing from this book is a detailed examination of chiropractors and self-styled "nutritionists" and their roles in MediScams, for example. The reason is that it would take an entire book to do justice to either subject. While many people benefit from the care of ethical chiropractors, it is also true that naïve as well as unscrupulous chiropractors are heavily involved in many MediScams, from bogus medical testing to prescribing worthless and overpriced dietary supplements. Many conventional medical practitioners would maintain that chiropractic as a whole is quackery. The basis of chiropractic is that "subluxations"—subtle misalignments of the vertebrae—are the cause of many pains and diseases. Yet there is no scientific evidence to show that chiropractic subluxations even exist. Rather than do a superficial job of addressing this topic in *MediScams,* I have chosen to leave it for another book.

Nutritionists are another group that would require their own book. I'm not referring here to registered dieticians, those who've earned the right to use the letters "R.D." after their names. These are legitimate professionals who work side by side with the medical community. I'm referring to the self-styled "experts" who use their guise as educated professionals simply as a marketing tool. To bolster their credibility, they often use initials like D.N.T. (for "doctor of nutritional therapy") or C.N.C. (for "certified nutritionist consultant"), or a myriad of other letters after their names. Usually, these are spurious mail-order credentials. Those who refer to themselves as "nutritionists" are often phonies who are simply out to sell you overpriced supplements that you most likely don't need.

This book opens with the tale of John Ronald "Butcher" Brown, who's been called "the worst doctor in America." I chose him as an example of the wanton and deplorable depths to which even people with legitimate medical training can sink. Yet I want to make clear that this is not a book about simple medical malpractice. All doctors can and do make mistakes, sometimes awful ones that kill patients—such is the price of being human. Likewise I want to make clear that I am not disparaging the medical profession as a whole. Were it not for competent, dedicated medical caregivers, I would not be alive to write these words.

Most doctors are kind, conscientious, and competent professionals who deliver the best care they can to their patients under what are often trying circumstances.

The problem is that the medical profession doesn't do nearly enough to weed out the bogus, incompetent, unethical, and alcohol- or drug-impaired physicians who are out among us practicing medicine. While there are many mechanisms available to stop bad doctors, ranging from hospital peer review committees to state medical licensing boards, the fact is that too often the medical community turns a blind eye to even the most obviously inept practitioners. By conservative estimates, one in ten medical doctors is practicing medicine while drug- or alcohol-impaired, yet fewer than one in one hundred doctors will be disciplined for it.

While we'll be looking at medical practitioners across the board in this book, two specialties have been singled out for special examination. The first is dentistry. I chose this profession because we don't normally associate dental treatments with scams. After all, a cavity is a cavity, right? Well, not always. The same tooth that one dentist says needs a simple filling for around $50, another may insist needs a root canal and a crown for around $1,250. And the reason for this difference may have more to do with greed than a difference of professional opinion. And, as we'll see, there are cults of dentists who favor diagnoses like "mercury amalgam toxicity" and "cavitational osteopathosis" that scientifically cannot be shown to exist.

The other specialty we'll be taking a close look at is plastic surgery. The economics of plastic surgery have created a gold mine for Medi-Scammers: Patients are willing to pay enormous sums of cash up front; in most cases there are no insurance or managed-care reviewers to challenge the need for the surgery; and most procedures are performed in private medical offices, away from the prying eyes of ethical medical professionals. As a result people from other medical specialties, often with minimal training, are now offering plastic surgery. Thus, we now have gynecologists offering liposuction, podiatrists (foot specialists) treating varicose veins, and dentists performing hair transplants. Even worse, there have been several instances of people billing themselves as "plastic sur-geons" who have had no medical training whatever. The result is not only wasted money but often tragic disfigurement and even death.

As I said earlier, the purpose of this book is not to disparage the medical community, but to make you a more educated and alert patient. The responsibility for seeking out appropriate and high-quality health care rests squarely on your own shoulders. We can't rely on our doctors to be right all the time. We must be prepared to do our own research about our treatment options and participate actively in our own medical care. We must recognize that quacks with no medical training are out there masquerading as doctors, so we should be prepared to check out a doctor's credentials thoroughly before entrusting our lives to his or her care. We need to keep our eyes and ears open, and make judgments for ourselves. Knowledge is power—in this case, the power to protect our money and our health from being victimized by a MediScam.

chapter 1

Every Patient's Nightmare

*Meet the Man Called "America's Worst Doctor"—
John Ronald "Butcher" Brown*

JOHN RONALD BROWN LOOKED more like a grandfatherly college professor than what he really was: a former surgeon who was so reckless, unethical, and grossly incompetent that he is now in prison for murder. He wore glasses that slid down his nose and had a double chin, and a belly hanging over his belt. He had large bags under his eyes, and his few remaining hairs were carefully combed across the top of his head in a vain attempt to hide his baldness. His lips were badly chapped and he sported long sideburns reminiscent of the 1950s. His hands trembled uncontrollably and his clothes were stained everywhere. He certainly didn't look like someone that any rational patient would want for a surgeon. But then, the patients who sought out the services of Dr. John Brown usually had plenty of problems even before he operated on them.

Gary Stovall and Steve Lindley, detectives with the police department of National City, California, a suburb of San Diego, conducted an interview with Brown on May 20, 1998. The detectives had found in a Holiday Inn room two receipts issued by Brown for $5,000 each. One was for "hospitalization" and the other for "surgery." They also found the dead body of one Philip Bondy. Bondy's identification indicated that he was a New York resident, seventy-nine years of age. The death bed showed evidence of a man in agony. There was blood everywhere and the corpse's face was frozen in a twisted mask of pain. Someone had cut off Bondy's left leg just above the knee, and the remaining stump had become inflamed and gangrenous. Who had amputated this man's leg and left him alone in a motel room? And why? That's what the detectives wanted to ask John Brown.

During their initial interrogation, the detectives could only get Brown to admit that he had spoken to Bondy a couple of times on the phone, that he had picked Bondy up at the San Diego airport and driven him to an undisclosed location, then returned him to the motel in National City where his body was found. Brown did, however, describe how to amputate a leg. Still, he wouldn't make any statement about what his role had been in Bondy's death. He admitted only to changing the bandage on Bondy's leg and noticing some blueness on the site of the amputation the day Bondy died.

It was immediately clear to Detectives Stovall and Lindley that Brown was hiding some very important details about Bondy's amputation and subsequent death. Brown was arrested two blocks from the station, having left the interrogation when the detectives were out of the room. The detectives' work had just begun.

According to a 1989 report by what is now the California Board of Medicine, this was not the first time John Brown had been questioned by authorities about his medical practices.

- In 1975 Brown was convicted for practicing medicine under a false name in Orange County, California.
- In 1977 his California medical license had been revoked following several findings of gross negligence involving transsexual surgeries, aiding unlicensed persons to practice medicine, and submitting false insurance claims.
- In 1979 a jury convicted Brown on twelve felony counts of prescribing controlled substances after his license had been revoked. He received a four-year probation in Los Angeles County.
- In 1983 Brown's petition to have his license restored was denied. Investigators for the California Board of Medicine found that Brown's

Alaska medical license had been revoked on November 19, 1982. And according to the San Diego County trial brief, his medical license had been revoked in Hawaii. He also had been thrown out of two hospitals in the Caribbean, on Dominica in 1980 and St. Lucia in 1981, for poor medical practices.

* In 1984 he was arrested in San Francisco for unlawfully representing himself as a licensed physician.

* In 1988 he pleaded guilty to five misdemeanor counts following his arrest on a failure-to-appear warrant. The judge had ordered that he not solicit patients, hold himself out as a physician, or practice medicine in California in any fashion, not even through a third-party intermediary.

Subsequent to the 1989 report, Brown was found guilty by a jury in 1990 of four felony counts involving the unlicensed practice of medicine in a manner likely to cause great bodily harm. He was sentenced to three years in a California state prison and ordered to pay restitution of $10,000. He was paroled in 1991.

AN UNIMPRESSIVE BACKGROUND

The man nicknamed "Butcher" Brown was born July 4, 1922, into a Mormon family. His father was a general practitioner. His childhood was, by his own admission, unremarkable, but he did manage to graduate from high school at the age of sixteen.

Brown received his bachelor's degree at the University of Utah in 1947. Just three months later, the same school issued his medical degree. He then moved to Los Angeles where he did his internship at Harbor General. He completed his internship training at Queen of Angels Hospital in Los Angeles. Brown then did general-surgery residencies at the University of Utah and Newark City Hospital, and a plastic-surgery residency at the Presbyterian Hospital in New York City. He admitted that he failed the general surgery oral examination twice and the plastic surgery oral examination three times. He never succeeded in passing either test to become board-certified in those specialties. Yet, because he was still considered board-eligible by virtue of having completed the specialty residencies, many hospitals allowed him to practice general surgery and plastic surgery in their facilities.

Brown had been married three times. His first wife ran off with a friend of his while he was in the army. His second wife died of breast cancer. He acquired his third wife in an arranged marriage in the Caribbean when she was just seventeen years old; Brown was fifty-nine. To this day, she remains devoted to Brown even though she divorced him while he was in prison in 1990. She would subsequently testify at Brown's trial that he taught her to read and write.

In addition to providing the usual general surgical procedures, Brown provided scalp-line relocation for people going bald. But his "specialty" was gender-reassignment surgery, which included breast implants and male genitalia removal for transsexuals, along with silicone injections, rib resectioning, liposuction, face-lifts and, on rare occasions, adding a penis to a woman who desired to become man.

Back when Brown was working in San Francisco, he employed a "Dr. James Spence." When asked, Brown would vouch for Spence's credentials as a doctor even though Spence was not licensed to practice medicine. At the time, Spence was on work furlough from prison; he had told Brown he was a veterinarian licensed in Africa.

California law requires a person who desires a gender change to meet extensive eligibility and readiness requirements, which include providing the surgeon with a psychological analysis and evidence that the candidate is rational, lucid, and understands the seriousness of such a decision. In addition, the candidate must live as a member of the opposite sex for one full year before receiving the surgery. Conventional practitioners will then perform the surgery under the same surgical safeguards as any other surgery in the U.S. While genital reconstruction surgery may cost up to $50,000 in the U.S. and $80,000 in Europe, if you elected to use Dr. John Brown, he would perform the surgery at Quintana Hospital in Tijuana,

Mexico, for less than $10,000. Despite what his brochure stated, you didn't have to worry about meeting the standard preliminary requirements. You simply walked through the door, put your money on the counter, and surgery would sometimes be performed that very day.

Such was the personal and professional caliber of the surgeon who met Philip Bondy at the San Diego airport on that fateful day in May 1998.

A RED-HERRING WITNESS

The person who discovered Bondy's body and called the police was Gregg Furth, Ph.D., a licensed psychologist from New York. In his initial statement to police, Furth identified himself as a good friend of Bondy's who had flown to San Diego the day before, due to concern over Bondy's condition. Furth told police that Bondy had called him on the evening of May 9. Bondy had said that he'd been in a traffic accident in Tijuana and had to have a leg amputated. On May 10 Furth hopped a plane and flew out to San Diego. He found Bondy quite dehydrated and hungry. Furth did not look at the stump, which was covered by the victim's clothing. He got food and drink for Bondy, and they talked until the evening hours. Furth and Bondy planned to fly back to New York together the next morning. However, when Furth entered Bondy's room around 8 A.M. the next morning, he discovered Bondy was dead and called hotel management. After he'd told his story, Furth flew back to New York.

Furth's account left unanswered many important questions. Why did Brown meet Bondy at the airport? And why did Brown perform the amputation and also collect $5,000 for the "hospitalization"? None of it made sense, so the detectives kept probing.

INVESTIGATING THE SURGEON FROM HELL

While Detectives Stovall and Lindley researched Brown's background, additional investigations were being conducted in other jurisdictions. For example, Los Angeles County had received a complaint from a patient on whom Brown had performed a breast-enlargement procedure that had consisted of nothing more than using a hypodermic syringe to inject silicone directly into the breasts. The injection holes had then been closed with superglue. One genetic female had received a face-lift, face peel, eye job, and breast implants. Her face had been left a scarred mess with a crooked smile despite Brown's three attempts to repair the damage. Her breasts had turned black and had to be removed.

Brown claimed he'd performed at least six hundred male-to-female surgeries. The results had not always been successful, to say the least. One transsexual complained that Brown had used a hairy scrotum to form the wall of her new vagina. The hairs continued to grow, resulting in recurrent infections. Another transsexual charged that she was excreting feces from her surgically made vagina. Following at least ten surgeries by Brown, yet another transsexual committed suicide: her mother said she had been despondent over the number of complications she had to endure. Many patients who had received gender-change surgeries from Brown complained about multiple malpractice experiences.

It was difficult for Detectives Stovall and Lindley to comprehend how someone like John Ronald Brown could have gotten away with so much for so long and still be practicing medicine anywhere.

More importantly to the case at hand, their investigations revealed there had been no major traffic accidents in Tijuana during the time of Bondy's visit to the city, let alone one that had resulted in a U.S. citizen having a leg amputated. Even more startling, the detectives found that Bondy had purchased a pair of crutches *before* his amputation surgery.

The detectives needed better answers from Furth, who had retained a San Diego attorney to represent him. After outlining Furth's likely testimony, the attorney negotiated an agreement in which Furth would turn state's evidence and be granted immunity for his testimony against Brown regarding the death of Philip Bondy. And Furth's testimony would prove the old adage that truth is, indeed, stranger than fiction.

A BIZARRE PSYCHOLOGICAL DISORDER

What follows is an excerpt from the district attorney's summary of the statement by Gregg Furth.

Gregg Furth is a Jungian Analyst, with a Ph.D. from Ohio State University. At the time of Mr. Bondy's death, Gregg Furth had known him for almost twenty-five years. They met in part due to the fact they both suffered from a fetish or paraphilia known as apotemnophilia. This fetish is also referred to as self-demand amputation, and involves primarily men who wish to have amputation of a lower extremity for psychological and sometimes sexual reasons. Dr. Furth stated he had been aware of wanting his own leg removed since his early childhood.

Over the course of many years, Dr. Furth and Philip Bondy became the best of friends. They continually researched the subjects of apotemnophilia and were constantly searching for a doctor who would remove a healthy limb, based on their psychological need for it. Dr. Furth co-authored a paper on apotemnophilia with Dr. John Money from Johns Hopkins University, a world-renowned and well-respected expert on the subject.

Brown and Furth made arrangements to meet in San Diego in April 1997. Brown told Furth the price for the surgery would be $3,000 and it would actually take place at a clinic in Tijuana. Furth sent Brown a $750 deposit check, which Brown deposited into his San Diego bank account. Furth flew out to San Diego around April, 1997. He stayed in a hotel near Shelter Island. Brown met him there and they discussed the procedure. At no time did Brown tell Furth that anyone other than himself would be performing the amputation. Brown did tell Furth that there would be a Mexican doctor who would assist him with anesthesia. At no time did Brown do any type of physical checkup on Furth, or ask to review any of his medical records or history. Furth purchased crutches in anticipation of losing his leg.

On the day of the surgery, Brown picked up Furth at his hotel and drove him into Mexico. At the clinic, Furth was introduced to a Mexican doctor. Shortly thereafter, Brown left them alone together. While waiting for Brown to return, the Mexican doctor began to question Furth about the reason for his amputation. When Furth began to explain that he did not have a physical health problem with his leg, but instead a mental problem, the doctor became enraged and began yelling at Furth. The doctor ultimately left the clinic, declining to participate in the surgery. Brown told Furth he would keep looking for someone else to assist him and would contact Furth when it was worked out. Furth returned to New York.

In early 1998, Brown called Furth from San Diego and told him that he had located another doctor to assist him with the anesthesia, but that the price would now be $10,000 for the surgery. Furth told Brown that he would have to get back to him because of the jump in price. Ultimately, Furth agreed to the new price and arrangements were made. The surgery was scheduled for late April 1998. As he had before, Furth kept Mr. Bondy informed of what was going on. Once again, Furth flew to San Diego for the surgery and met with Brown. On the day of the surgery, Brown picked up Furth. Furth gave Brown $9,250 in traveler's checks (having already paid $750 the year before), but he only endorsed half of them. On the way to the clinic, Brown stopped at a bank in San Ysidro, leaving Furth in the car. Once at the clinic, Dr. Furth met the new anesthesiologist. Almost immediately, he began to have second thoughts about going through with the surgery. Brown tried to convince him to go ahead and take some sedatives to help him calm down, but Furth refused. Furth declined to proceed. Brown was not happy about this change in circumstance.

Somehow, either Furth or Brown suggested that they call Philip to see if he wanted to take Furth's place. Furth placed the call, telling his friend that he was not able to go through with the surgery. When asked if he wanted to take his place, Mr. Bondy replied something close to, "You bet I will!" Furth then gave the phone to Brown and listened as Brown made arrangements to operate on Bondy approximately two weeks later. Again, Furth stated that all negotiations between he and Bondy as well as those he overheard while Brown was talking on the phone to Bondy were that Brown was the surgeon who would be performing the amputation. After the phone call, Brown gave Furth back $4,250 worth of traveler's checks which he had stuffed in his sock. He told Furth that Furth could negotiate with the other doctor to try to get the other $5,000 back. Furth decided to leave the money to be applied toward Bondy's surgery and then get his $5,000 back from his friend.

On May 7th, 1998, Philip Bondy flew to San Diego and checked into the Holiday Inn.

The rest of the story you know.

Approximately two hundred people in the world at any given time are afflicted with apotemnophilia. A person suffering from this condition believes he or she can only become attractive by losing a limb. It's illegal for a physician to remove a healthy limb, so when people with this psychological disorder ask licensed surgeons to cut off a leg or arm, the normal response is a psychiatric referral. No responsible physician would even consider cutting off someone's leg without substantial medical justification. But then, "responsible physician" is a label few people would apply to John Ronald Brown, M.D.

A CHARGE OF MURDER

Christina Stanley, M.D., the San Diego County deputy medical examiner, performed an autopsy on Philip Bondy on May 12, 1998, approximately twenty-five hours after his body was found at the Holiday Inn. The autopsy findings concluded that Bondy died of gas gangrene of the left leg that had been caused by an unnecessary surgical procedure. Specifically Stanley said, "In consideration of the reported scene investigations, autopsy findings and circumstances surrounding the death, as currently understood, the medically unnecessary amputation, which lead [sic] to the death, was performed without standard medical preoperative, perioperative or postoperative care. For these reasons, the manner of death is classified as homicide."

Meanwhile, the detectives continued their investigation. They obtained a search warrant and combed Brown's apartment. He was a bachelor who had no knack for keeping an orderly home. The detectives found bloodstains in the apartment which would eventually be found to contain DNA from five different individuals, according to prosecutors. The detectives also found towels covered with what appeared to be blood, soaking in a bathtub filled with water and bleach. In the bedroom they found what appeared to be blood on the bed's sheets, mattress, and pillowcases. Inside Brown's travel bags were a variety of surgical tools, blood-soaked towels, and tubes labeled "superglue" and "superglue remover." Gauze, bandages, and drugs were everywhere. In Brown's car they found a box of surgical tools, medical supplies, and surgical masks on the floor of his trunk. Could Brown actually have been performing surgeries and attending patients in his apartment and vehicle?

Detectives also found numerous videotapes Brown had made of his surgeries. These would prove to be very damaging during his trial. In two instances one could hear patients screaming in pain as he cut into them without administering sufficient anesthesia. In an exposé for the TV program *Inside Edition,* the well-respected California surgeon Alan Gaynor reviewed Brown's videotaped work. Gaynor appeared visibly shaken by the horrific conditions under which Brown operated on patients. The program reported that some surgeries even took place in garages. For his part, Brown stated that the *Inside Edition* piece had slandered him.

Enter Stacy L. Running, San Diego County deputy district attorney. Running is an attractive blue-eyed blonde who could be a fashion model just as easily as the hard-hitting prosecutor of murderers she really is. It was Running's job to prosecute Brown, who had been charged with the murder of Philip Bondy, along with nine counts of the unlawful practice of medicine causing risk and great bodily harm between May 20, 1995, and April 30, 1998. To make the murder charge stick, Running would have to prove Brown had had a history of reckless behavior as a medical practitioner.

A MURDERER IS FINALLY PUT AWAY

The trial of John Ronald Brown began on September 23, 1999. Deputy D.A. Running systematically walked the court through Brown's history of malpractice and reckless indifference to his patients' welfare, and his repeated refusals to stop practicing medicine even after his license had been revoked. One of the prosecution's exhibits was a copy of Brown's own promotional brochure for transsexual surgeries.

Brown's defense was that he had believed that it was legal for him to work under a licensed physician in Mexico. Therefore, he had been unaware he was breaking any laws. He also argued that death on the surgical table is a fact of life. If prosecutors charged every surgeon who lost a patient with murder, there wouldn't be any surgeons left—so why should he be singled out and prosecuted for murder because a patient died from an unexpected infection? He also attempted to convince the jury that he was a humanitarian helping people who had been ignored by established medicine; if not for him, these people would have led horrible, empty lives. The jury didn't buy his arguments, or his amiable, grandfatherly demeanor: Brown was found guilty and sentenced to fifteen years to life in prison.

After he had lost his California medical license in 1977, Brown said that God had told him to take care of the needs of "his children," the transsexuals. Now, in prison, John Ronald Brown says he cannot help people directly so he is working on the design of a hyperthermia chamber that will, he says, cure cancer, AIDS, and genital herpes. Each night Brown prays God will release him from prison so he can go back to helping others.

For her part, Deputy D.A. Running hopes that Brown never leaves prison alive. After all, she points out, nobody knows how many other people suffered death or disfigurement at his hands. And she's convinced that if he were released from prison today, he would be killing and maiming people tomorrow. Says Running, "I'd be afraid for others. If he got out, he'd be operating the very next day. He believes that he is doing people a service."

PATIENT BEWARE!

John Ronald Brown is just one of the many MediScammers we'll be taking a hard look at in this book. As I said in the Introduction, most doctors are competent, conscientious, and dedicated professionals who deliver quality medical care to their patients. This book certainly is not intended to do a disservice to them. But, for a variety of reasons that will be explored in future chapters, the medical community is ineffective in protecting the public from bad, bogus, or unscrupulous physicians and other promoters of unnecessary and sometimes downright dangerous "treatments"—what I call MediScams. Fortunately most MediScams follow predictable and recognizable promotional strategies that set them apart from legitimate medical therapies. It's up to us, the consumers of medical care, to become more aware of MediScams and how they operate so that we can recognize a rip-off before we sacrifice our money, or our health, on bad or fraudulent treatments. And that's what this book is all about. After all, the MediScammer's worst enemy is a wary and educated patient.

chapter 2

A Brief History of MediScams

From Snake Oil to Cancer Quackery

MEDICAL FRAUD, QUACKERY, AND bogus cures have been around as long as there has been the desire to cure illness. In fact, the term "quack" is short for *quacksalvers,* the Renaissance peddlers who sold mercury (quicksilver)-based salves. During that time, mercury compounds were the treatment for syphilis and were also used as diuretics and purgatives. The quacksalvers claimed their salves cured nearly all known diseases.

A brief review of the history of American quackery proves true the old adage that the more things change, the more they stay the same. Although quacks have grown more sophisticated, their basic claims and tactics have changed little since the Renaissance. They still exploit the niche between what the patient needs and wants, and what reputable medicine can deliver. They still spew out whatever the patient wants to hear, regardless of the facts. And they still make money, robbing the sick of time and resources better spent seeking legitimate treatment or preparing for the inevitable.

EARLY AMERICAN QUACKERY

One of the earliest recorded quacks in America was Nicholas Knopp of the Massachusetts Bay colony. In 1630 he was given a choice of paying a fine of five pounds or being publicly whipped for selling "a water of no worth nor value" as a cure for scurvy. He was only the first of many to follow. At a time when few legitimate medications of any value existed, colonists were easy prey for hucksters who offered every form of cure-all. And it wasn't always just their elixirs that were bogus: The town of Chester, Pennsylvania, jailed a snake-oil salesman by the name of Charles Hamilton after discovering that Hamilton was in fact a woman. Another colonial huckster by the name of Francis Torres sold "Chinese stones" as a cure for toothache, cancer, and the bites of mad dogs and rattlesnakes. The "stones" were apparently shaped from deer antler then burned in hot embers.

Back then, of course, it was difficult for even an educated person to distinguish between quackery and what passed for "legitimate" medicine. One of the most respected pioneers of American medicine, Dr. Benjamin Rush, employed bleeding and purging to treat victims of the yellow fever epidemic of 1793. Rush was also one of the three well-respected physicians who administered care to a dying George Washington. Their treatments included bleeding, blistering, and the administration of calomel, a powder containing mercurous chloride. Although this was considered state-of-the-art health care at the time, it almost certainly hastened Washington's death.

CASHING IN ON SCIENCE

Quacks are forever in search of new gimmicks and have known since the beginning of modern scientific investigation that a good way to promote their latest "miracle cure" is to link it with an authentic scientific discovery. Again, given the state of medicine prior to the twentieth century, the boundaries between quackery and legitimate medical science were often fuzzy at best. For example, in the mid-1700s, Christian Kratzenstein found that his patients showed a quickened pulse when exposed to newly discovered electrical currents. He went on to use electrical currents to treat rheumatism, malignant fever, and the plague. Although this treatment was totally useless, so were almost all the other treatments then in use for these conditions.

As the use of electricity spread, so did the number and variety of supposedly curative electrical devices. Around 1900, *Cosmopolitan* magazine ran ads for the "Electropoise," which allegedly placed "the body in condition to absorb oxygen from the lungs." The same person also sold the Oxydonor, which "forced oxygen into the system" and claimed to be beneficial for no fewer than eighty-six diseases.

The 1920s saw the development and marketing of the "I-on-a-co" and "Theranoid" body coils. Both devices were essentially solenoids consisting of eighteen-inch coils of several hundred feet of insulated wire covered with simulated leather, and looking rather like a horse collar. The device was placed around the patient's midsection and plugged into the household current several times a day for "treatments" that would allegedly cure every known disease.

Around the same time, a physician by the name of Albert Abrams was inventing a number of gadgets. One of his machines, the "Dynamizer," was based on Abrams' claim that every disease had a signature electronic vibration that could be measured. The "Electronic Reactions of Abrams" or ERA readings measured by the Dynamizer could then be used to pinpoint where the disease was in a patient. This approach to medicine was endorsed by the Jehovah's Witnesses religious community until the early 1960s when the church's oversight group, the Watchtower Society, finally realized that it was quackery.

Other scientific findings also engendered quack cures. The mid-nineteenth century discovery that infectious diseases were caused by microbes inspired Texas gardener William Radam to create his "Microbe Killer," a tonic that he claimed destroyed microbes and cured disease. The government found it contained mostly water, with less than one percent hydrochloric and sulfuric acids and red wine. The Curies' discovery of radium and early experiments with radiation inspired someone going by the name of "Dr. Rupert Wells" to advertise and sell Radol, a "radium impregnated" fluid that would cure cancer in all forms, locations, and stages. *Collier's* magazine reported that Radol "contains exactly as much radium as dishwater does, and is about as efficacious in cancer or consumption [tuberculosis]."

The end of World War II saw an astounding leap in technology. Our understanding of radar led to the development of microwave ovens. Rockets made space exploration possible. Television became commonplace, and computers opened an entirely new horizon to our thinking. Reputable medicine benefited from a host of new diagnostic and therapeutic technologies, raising the hopes and expectations of patients everywhere. And the quacks were trailing close behind, always ready to make a quick buck off the desperate and gullible.

In 1958, a West German physician by the name of Reinhold Voll combined Chinese acupuncture theory with differences in the electrical conductivity of the skin to produce the "Electroacupuncture According to Voll" (EAV) procedure, also known as electrodiagnosis, electrodermal screening, and BioResonance Therapy, among other names. A number of devices were spawned by this procedure, going by names like Accupath 1000, Biotron, Computron, and so on. The basic idea is that the patient holds one electrode as the practitioner applies another electrode to various acupuncture points on the skin. The device measures the electrical resistance between the electrodes, and from this the practitioner "diagnoses" the patient's condition and selects the appropriate homeopathic remedy. Alternatively, sometimes the device itself is used to treat the patient's condition. Although the Food and Drug Administration (FDA) has cracked down on many of these devices and banned their importation, the simple fact is that the quacks are able to mutate new variations of the EAV devices faster than the FDA can identify and stop them.

Dubious medical devices continue to proliferate. Peruse almost any popular magazine or watch late-night television and you'll be bombarded with ads for devices that are alleged to cure acne, remove "cellulite" without exercise or diet, or even enlarge a favorite part of your anatomy. Hundreds of such gadgets have been collected and put on display in the Museum of Questionable Medical Devices in Minneapolis, Minnesota, by its curator, Bob McCoy.

THE RISE AND FALL OF PATENT MEDICINES

Patent medicine is almost synonymous with quackery, especially in the American West. The term "patent medicine" originated in England and referred to "patents of royal favor" that kings granted to their bootmakers, tailors, and medicine makers. By definition, true patent medicines revealed their ingredients on their labels as a condition of maintaining their patent on that formulation. The so-called "patent medicines" produced in America were actually proprietary drugs in which the unique shape and color of the bottles along with the label designs were protected by trademark. The actual ingredients within the bottles, however, were kept secret—a practice that only added to the medicine's mystique. "Patent medicine" became a misused term due to the lack of distinction between patented and unpatented medicines in ads and on store shelves. Before the American Revolution, commonly imported English patent medicines included Anderson's Scots Pills, Godfrey's Cordial, Dr. John Hooper's Female Pills, Dr. Bateman's Pectoral Drops, and Robert Turlington's Balsam of Life. Dr. Bateman's drops were said to cure gout, rheumatism, jaundice, stone, asthma, colds, rickets, and melancholy.

Probably the first documented advertisement for a nostrum (defined in *Webster's Ninth New Collegiate Dictionary* as "a medicine of secret composition recommended by its preparer but usually without scientific proof of its effectiveness") was an October 4, 1708, ad in the *Boston News-Letter* for Daffy's Elixir Salutis for colic and griping (abdominal cramps). By the 1750s, advertisements for English nostrums appeared in papers published throughout the colonies. These products were sold not only by apothecaries but by postmasters, goldsmiths, grocers, hairdressers, and others.

By the middle of the eighteenth century, there was a great demand for British patent medicines, and enterprising apothecaries began refilling the familiar-looking bottles with their own formulas and selling them to unsuspecting customers. This practice increased during the American Revolution when bottles could not be imported from England. After the war, price undercutting of British-made nostrums encouraged sales of domestic versions of popular medicines.

In the late eighteenth century, Samuel Lee Jr. of Windham, Connect-icut, became the first American to patent a medicine. His "Bilious Pills" were recommended for treating yellow fever, jaundice, dysentery, dropsy (edema), worms, and "female complaints." Three years later, Samuel H. P. Lee from New London, Connecticut, patented his own version of "Bilious Pills," which contained mercury-laden calomel. Both brands of Bilious Pills proved to be immensely popular.

One of the most successful nineteenth-century nostrum makers was Thomas Dyott. In the 1810s, Dyott was making a line of "family reme-dies" named for a Dr. Robertson who was supposedly an Edinburgh physician and Dyott's grandfather. Even after a Philadelphia physician discovered that no Dr. Robertson had practiced in Edinburgh for nearly two centuries, Dyott continued to sell Dr. Robertson's Infallible Worm Destroying Lozenges and other concoctions. His sales increased after he took on the title of "Doctor of Medicine" and invented a résumé that included work in London, the West Indies, and Philadelphia. Dyott advertised in daily papers and rural weeklies and later started agencies in New York, Cincinnati, New Orleans, and other cities.

By the 1840s, the population had moved westward and farther away from where goods were manufactured. More and more supplies, includ-ing specific patent medicines, were moved by railroad and by post to meet the demands of a growing nation.

Newspapers were also started up everywhere, and in all those news-papers appeared advertisements for—you guessed it—patent medicines. In fact, just before the Civil War, about one-half of *all* advertising, not just in newspapers, was for medicines. The biggest advertiser, James C. Ayer, published ads for his Cherry Pectoral, and later, pills and sarsaparillas, in every newspaper across the country. Sixteen million copies of various editions of his *American Almanacs* were being printed every year. In 1889, he printed almanacs and pamphlets in twenty-one languages for distri-bution around the world.

Commercial almanacs began running ads for patent medicines in the 1820s. By 1844, patent-medicine makers were publishing their own almanacs, complete with astronomical and astrological data, advice for the farmer and housewife, jokes, and the inevitable sales pitch. These free almanacs were delivered to druggists and shopkeepers (who were charged a nominal amount to cover shipping costs), then placed on counters or distributed by hand to millions of families. In some cases, the almanac was the only form of literature in a household, and it was often used as an informal textbook.

During the Civil War, Hostetter's Bitters was promoted to the Union Army as "a positive protective against the fatal maladies of the Southern swamps." The war itself hurt some northern nostrum makers who lost their southern markets. However, these markets expanded rapidly after the Civil War to include thousands of soldiers with malaria, wounds, and chronic ailments who had come to rely on patent medicines.

MEDICINE SHOWS: BE ENTERTAINED AND CURED

Medicine shows, leading forms of entertainment and health care providers from about 1870 to 1920, were at their peak during the last two decades of the nineteenth century. Advertisements for medicine shows and patent medicines sprang up in brochures on drugstore counters, paintings on barns, in almanacs, religious and country weekly newspapers, daily newspapers, and even in the back pages of popular novels. Featured in the medicine show was the pitchman, usually a self-appointed doctor who often wore a top hat and frock coat and wandered from town to town supported by his cast of ex-circus performers, traveling theater troupes, vaudeville acts, and minstrel shows. Snake oil, especially rattle-snake oil, was taken very seriously by patrons of medicine shows. Of course, snake oil didn't come from snakes; it was often a mixture of white gasoline and wintergreen oil.

Manufacturers of patent medicines sometimes put together their own touring companies to market their products. Perhaps the biggest medicine show ever was assembled by John E. Healy and "Texas Charley" Bigelow, who formed the Kickapoo Indian Medicine Company in 1881. Their traveling shows each had about a dozen players, white and Indian, who promoted various products, including Kickapoo Indian Oil ("the Quick Cure for All Pains"), Kickapoo Indian Salve ("Healing, Purifying, Soothing"), and Kickapoo Indian Worm Killer ("requires no After-Physic"). During the 1880s, seventy-five or so Kickapoo shows might be on tour at the same time, with an occasional stationary show with up to one hundred performers.

THE WAR ON PATENT MEDICINES

Patients who took patent medicines often did feel better—not because they were "cured" of anything but because the medicines frequently contained powerful narcotics, including morphine, heroin, cocaine, opium, as well as alcohol in amounts that sometimes approached that of whiskey. Another problem additive was acetanilide, an effective pain reliever that is toxic when used regularly. And it was the widespread use of such ingredients that would contribute to the downfall of patent medicines.

The attack on patent medicines began soon after the Civil War when many patients found themselves addicted to the narcotic-laced medicines. In 1884 the Association of Official Agricultural Chemists began testing tonics for alcohol, "soothing" syrups for morphine, and headache powders for acetanilide, then publishing their results in pamphlets. The *American Agriculturist* magazine excluded objectionable nostrum advertising, and other popular magazines such as the *Ladies' Home Journal* waged a campaign against patent medicines. Beginning in 1905, Samuel Hopkins Adams wrote a series of articles for *Collier's* magazine called "The Great American Fraud" in which he revealed the high levels of alcohol in patent medicines and discussed the bogus claims made as well as the enormous profits reaped by the manufacturers.

In the decades preceding the Pure Food and Drug Act of 1906, many legislative measures that dealt with mislabeling and adulteration of food and drugs were introduced but not passed by Congress. Dr. Harvey Wiley, chief chemist of the Department of Agriculture and writer of the act, partially blamed the failure of earlier measures to pass on those who thought it would terminate their lucrative business practices. And patent medicines were indeed lucrative: In 1900 alone, 2,026 patent-medicine companies had a combined production valued at $59,611,335. Five years later, a drug trade journal listed the names of over 28,000 patent medicines.

The Pure Food and Drug Act of 1906 required that the amount of specific narcotic drugs, as well as alcohol, must always be named on the label or package, and that the actual amount of the stated ingredient must match this claim. However, the law was found to be inadequate, as demonstrated by the case of a Dr. Johnson, who was prosecuted for selling a worthless cancer treatment. Johnson won his case because he had fulfilled the labeling requirements.

The American Medical Association (AMA) launched its own campaign against quackery when Dr. Arthur J. Cramp became involved with the *Journal of the American Medical Association (JAMA)*. *JAMA* began publishing items on quackery and health fraud on a regular basis, and also reprinted 150,000 copies of Adams' articles on quackery in *Collier's* in booklet form for distribution to individuals and libraries.

In 1911 the first edition of the book *Nostrums and Quackery* was published by the AMA. This edition was later enlarged, and within the next decade a second volume was issued. The AMA also attacked certain companies and products in *JAMA*, citing results from chemical analyses showing their products were bogus or mislabeled. *JAMA* attempted to verify "patient testimonials" used by such manufacturers, often finding them to have been falsified, unreliable, or forged. *JAMA* also discussed manufacturing costs, revealing in one case that a medicine that cost twenty-four cents a bottle to manufacture was being sold for $5. Even more important in the war against patent medicines, however, was the passage of the Harrison Federal Narcotics Act of 1914. This act restricted the use of narcotics in medicines except where prescribed by a physician in the course of professional practice. Patent medicines were exempt from the licensing and tax provisions of the act as long as they limited themselves to "preparations and remedies which do not contain more than two grains of opium, or more than one-fourth of a grain of morphine, or more than one-eighth of a grain of heroin in one avoirdupois ounce." With this step, many patent medicines suddenly lost their allure.

Despite the efforts of the AMA and others, patent medicines continued to sell well in the 1920s and 1930s. Not surprisingly, tonics containing alcohol were especially popular during Prohibition. During this time, safety continued to be an issue, and it's estimated that thirty-five to fifty thousand Americans suffered severe reactions to patent medicines in the 1920s. One of the most tragic cases involved a compound marketed under the name "Elixir Sulfanilamide." Sulfanilamide, one of the first truly effective antibiotics, had been called a miracle medicine by the press, and nothing was wrong with the drug itself. The problem was that a chemist had used the solvent diethylene glycol in formulating the elixir. The chemist had found the solvent acceptable in appearance, fragrance, and flavor, but overlooked one critical detail—diethylene glycol is poisonous to humans. Almost two thousand pints were distributed, but the solvent was not listed on a single label. The FDA was able to take action only because all "elixirs" were supposed to contain alcohol and this one didn't. An estimated 107 people, many of them children, died painful deaths before the agency was able to track down and recover the remaining bottles. The chemist who created the elixir committed suicide and the company owner, a doctor, paid a fine of $26,100.

Medical fraud became so prolific that in 1927 the Bureau of the Chief Post Office Inspector formed a special unit of inspectors who investigated quackery cases and gathered evidence to support criminal or civil prosecution against the promoters.

But what finally killed off the fraudulent patent medicines was the Food, Drug and Cosmetic Act of 1938. As it pertained to patent medicines, the act required that drug companies prove scientifically that a product was safe before it could be sold. The act also stated that it wasn't necessary for the FDA to prove fraud in order "to stop a manufacturer from making untrue statements about a drug's effectiveness." The act further specified that the common names and quantities of all active ingredients, especially habit-forming narcotics and other potent drugs, had to be listed on the label.

The end of Prohibition in 1933 had already eroded the allure of alcohol-bearing elixirs. As a result of the Food, Drug and Cosmetic Act of 1938, there could be no more "secret" formulas and no more false or unsubstantiated claims about a medicine's potential benefits. Finally exposed to the light of day, the patent-medicine industry—like the bloodsucking vampires of legend—began to wither away.

THE CAMPAIGN AGAINST HEALTH FRAUD

With the 1938 Food, Drug and Cosmetic Act in place, the FDA began a campaign to make all medications and cosmetics safe. The first product seizure under the new law was of an eyelash beautifier that had left chemical burns on the eyes of an Ohio woman, as reported in the *Detroit Free Press* on July 23, 1938.

During the 1940s, a number of seizures of products occurred, such as laxatives which contained dangerous drugs. And the FDA also was able to remove hazardous devices, such as pessaries (intrauterine devices to induce abortion or prevent conception), dilators, nipple shields, electric insoles, eye massagers, and bust developers, which proliferated on the West Coast. But the FDA had problems combating quackery because many of its lawsuits were contested, and it had limited resources to pursue these costly cases.

The AMA, Post Office, FDA, and the Better Business Bureau (BBB) joined forces to go after the most blatant cases of quackery. Diabetes was a favorite of quacks because of the short life expectancy of its victims and the attractiveness of a quick cure over the standard treatment which included a diet restricted in both quantity and types of food.

Dr. Charles Frederick Kaadt was a quack who offered a "cure" for diabetes that didn't use insulin or a diet. Sold by mail, his $5 treatment was a bottle containing a twenty-day supply of his special tonic. He was first cited for misbranding in 1932, but he simply rewrote the bottle's label to omit the claim that it was a cure for diabetes. He ran into problems again when the FDA reported to the Post Office that Kaadt's venture might be fraudulent and he shouldn't be allowed to use the mail. The case was eventually dismissed, but to avoid trouble Kaadt stopped using the mails and instead insisted that his patients come to his institute in South Whitley, Indiana, for a three-day treatment. Hundreds of new patients arrived every day. The workload was so overwhelming that Kaadt's physician brother, Peter, closed his Oregon practice and joined Charles.

In May 1946 a letter of complaint from the president of the American Diabetes Association was sent to the AMA. The BBB, which had been collecting information about the Kaadt brothers, sent an agent to investigate. Pretending to be a potential patient, the agent was hurriedly diagnosed as a diabetic and sold medicine for home treatment. The "medicine" proved to be nothing more than a mixture of vinegar and saltpeter.

The BBB petitioned the Indiana Board of Medical Registration and Examination to revoke Charles Kaadt's medical license. Eventually the board met, and Charles agreed to the cancellation of his license even before all the evidence had been presented. Peter Kaadt closed the clinic after Charles left, but reopened a private practice for diabetes sufferers in the same building. The board went after Peter's license and won, but lost on appeal. Peter had another year to sell his saltpeter-and-vinegar "medicine" before the Supreme Court reversed the decision and revoked his license for good.

The FDA also had been gathering evidence against the Kaadt brothers, and indicted them on seven counts of violating the 1938 Act. They were convicted in April of 1948 but, due to poor health, they were each fined $7,000 and sentenced to only four years in prison. Peter died before his four years were up. Charles served his term and died soon afterward.

The U.S. Postal Inspectors gained another quack-busting tool in 1952 when the wire-fraud statute was enacted. This statute, patterned after mail fraud laws, covered the use of interstate wire, radio, or telephone communications for the purpose of carrying out a scheme to

defraud. This statute has been used more and more over the years as telemarketing is often used in conjunction with mail fraud.

Today, the FDA continues its fight against quack cures, although its
current efforts focus mostly on public education and awareness. In large
part this is due to the enormous difficulty and cost of prosecuting
offenders. Back in 1986, the cost was some $200,000 to $300,000 per
criminal prosecution. And with the advent of the Internet, tracking
down quacks is harder than ever, especially since many of them now
operate outside the U.S. borders.

OLD SCAMS, NEW SUCKERS

In my view, the hallmark of a truly successful MediScam is that it creates
a cult following that allows it to outlive its inventor. Homeopathic medicines are probably the best known and most widely practiced Medi-
Scams in existence. Despite FDA efforts to eradicate it, Laetrile still has
its users and defenders. Likewise, a search of the Internet finds that there
are several sites that defend and promote the "electronic reactions" of
Abrams. Some would argue that the "bioresonance" therapies popular in
Europe and discussed in chapter 7 are nothing more than a variation of
the ERA.

Another fascinating MediScammer whose nonsensical theories live
on is Dale Alexander, whose book *Arthritis and Common Sense,* first published in 1949, claimed to have found a cure for arthritis. Alexander
reportedly bought a bogus Ph.D. from the Stanley College of the Spoken
Word, a diploma mill in England, instantly transforming himself into
"Dr. Alexander." With his newfound credentials, he wrote several books.
The *Los Angeles Times* listed one of his books in the "Top 100 Books of
the Century," and *Publisher's Weekly* nominated his book about a cure for
arthritis for "The Book of the Generation," according to the Cancer
Control Society flyer for the 13th Annual Cancer Convention in 1985.

According to Alexander's own story, his interest in arthritis started
one night when he heard a squeaking sound coming from his mother

who was afflicted with arthritis. He reasoned that human joints, like mechanical joints, required lubrication. Thus, he claimed to find the answer to cure arthritis. All the afflicted had to do was drink cod-liver oil.

He claimed that, after giving his mother cod-liver oil daily for a short period of time, her symptoms completely disappeared. He also claimed that he spent ten years researching the scientific literature before writing his bestselling book on the subject.

Just taking the oil was not enough, of course. The patient had to understand the dietary rules so the cod-liver oil would "bypass the liver" and go directly to the joints. If you wanted to know the rules you had to read *Arthritis and Common Sense*. You could purchase his book along with his special brand of cod-liver oil, which he claimed came in three flavors, "icky, yucky, and lousy."

Alexander wrote that arthritis sufferers should lubricate their joints by eating foods rich in dietary oils but should avoid acids such as grapefruit or lemon juices which cut the oils, drying out the body. He warned that arthritics should be wary of drinking water, which doesn't mix with oils. Yet his sample menus were well-balanced and nutritional.

Arthritis and Common Sense remained on the bestseller list for forty-two weeks and from time to time ranked number one. It was reported at the time that over half a million people had tried the cod-liver formula. Dr. Alexander appeared as a guest on TV's *The Arthur Godfrey Show* and gave speeches all over the U.S. One speech he gave in Florida had over 6,000 attendees.

Although Alexander claimed to have studied pre-med at Trinity College and taken courses at Columbia University, in truth he took one high-school-level course at Trinity, and studied at Columbia a few weeks before dropping out, according to a 1957 *Life* magazine article by Robert Wallace.

It was not the FDA or the FBI that came after Dale Alexander. It was the Federal Trade Commission (FTC), charging him with false advertising on the basis that his suggestions wouldn't cure any kind of arthritis. The Arthritis and Rheumatism Foundation's medical and scientific committee concluded the book was full of erroneous information and contrary to scientific knowledge to state that joints were lubricated by oils or fats consumed. They called it a dangerous book.

So why did thousands of people swear that Alexander's dietary formula worked? According to the Arthritis and Rheumatism Foundation, there were a few good reasons. The first is that many who took the oil did not have arthritis in the first place. The second reason is that, at any given point, approximately one-third of rheumatoid arthritis sufferers are entering a natural period of remission, another one-third are entering a period of relapse, and about one-third feel "about the same"—thus, if anyone gives any kind of treatment to any group of arthritis sufferers, around one-third are going to report improvement. That equals thousands of believers.

Once Alexander cured arthritis, he turned his attention to cancer. He believed that cancer was caused by "bypassing the saliva." This problem occurred, he said, because people drink carbonated sodas and Perrier water. These beverages then cause a pre-cancerous condition he called "greening of the elbow." He actually said the person's elbow would turn green! Sound far-fetched? Remember, this was coming from the man who had been credited with finding the cure for arthritis. Like Dr. Albert Abrams, Alexander had the credibility to carry off a MediScam on little more than his word alone.

In the end Alexander probably did not hurt anyone with his cod-liver oil. He may have been well intentioned but, like so many snake-oil salesmen, the only thing he really came up with was a cure for personal poverty.

Arthritis and Common Sense is still in print. I found it being sold through an online bookstore, where it received an Average Customer Review of five stars, their highest rating. One online reviewer with rheumatoid arthritis wrote in December 1999 that "Dale Alexander is one of the few M.D.'s who has actually taken the time to research the impact nutrition has on arthritis, and it is significant." And so the MediScam lives on.

WHY SCAMS CONTINUE

At first thought, we might be tempted to believe that modern medicine would be able to squeeze quacks out of business. After all, why buy a bogus cure when a real one is there for the asking? The reality, sadly, is that modern medicine has simply created more niches than ever for the quacks and MediScammers to fill. In the first place, science and medicine have raised patient expectations faster than they have been able to fulfill them. If we can put a man on the moon, the reasoning goes, surely we should be able to cure cancer and AIDS! The fact that we really can't creates a gigantic vacuum in patient expectations that quacks are only too eager to fill. Another opening for the quacks is created by the fact that effective medical treatments are often unpleasant and painful. "Why undergo cancer surgery and chemotherapy," the quack asks, "when instead you can take my pills or injections and receive the same result with little pain or discomfort?" Quacks will continue to flourish as long as they are able to convince patients that they have the "secret" to a safer, simpler, and more effective treatment than legitimate physicians have to offer.

It's fair to say that some vitamins and food supplements have become the successors to patent medicines. Like patent medicines, they are heavily advertised and often make extravagant and false claims. And their manufacturers are raking in the profits from those whom they confuse and defraud. Although supplement manufacturers are prohibited from making unproven claims in advertising or on product labels, they often break the law by making such claims in "informational" pamphlets or in their sales pitches.

In the mid-1980s, the FDA went after General Nutrition Corporation's (GNC) marketing of evening primrose oil and won. Even though GNC claimed the product was sold as a dietary supplement, their sales literature and salespeople claimed that this product could cure arthritis, hypertension, and multiple sclerosis (MS). GNC pled guilty to selling a misbranded drug and was fined $10,000.

Another good example of how things haven't changed much since the late nineteenth century would be the marketing of mineral water. In

1996, the U.S. Postal Service sued Aerobic Life Industries, Inc., for fraud, alleging that the company had marketed their "Aerobic 07" mineral water as a remedy, cure, or treatment for arthritis, diabetes, ulcers, MS, Alzheimer's, and AIDS, among other ailments. As with the patent medicines of yore, the sales pitch included a complete guarantee, testimonials from satisfied patients, a scientific "theory" to explain how the water worked such miracles, and recommendations by reputed medical experts. In 1996, Aerobic Life Industries was ordered to cease and desist from making false claims about their mineral water.

The government's legal and educational battle against quackery continues. Organizations like the American Diabetes Association, the American Cancer Society, the AMA, and dozens of others provide information about valid medical treatment options and try to steer the public away from false cures. Yet the outrageous claims made by advocates of bogus devices, worthless medications, and needless dietary supplements constantly bombard us. As long as there is a disease that can't be cured by reputable medicine, there will always be a MediScammer offering a bogus therapy that promises to "cure" the disease—for a price. Too often, that price is not just money but the patient's health or even life.

As an investigative reporter I've confronted my share of MediScams. Many of them will be described in later chapters of this book. Some of these scams were so blatantly fraudulent, it's hard to believe anyone could fall for them. But they were the exceptions. Most were clever enough that even some well-educated professionals were taken in by them. Just as medicine has grown more sophisticated over the years, so have the quacks and MediScammers. In fact, some MediScammers are themselves well-trained physicians with impeccable medical and scientific credentials. And many well-meaning people actually *believe* in the therapies or products they sell.

As consumers, we have to be aware of how prevalent MediScams really are, and know that they may operate on every level of health care, from the finest teaching hospital to your next-door neighbor who sells vitamins through a multilevel marketing program. We have to be prepared to do some of our own research. The appendix of this book offers a number of resources, including a list of telephone numbers and Web site addresses for organizations providing health information as well as others specifically dedicated to exposing bogus medical treatments, such as Quackwatch, the National Council for Reliable Health Information (NCRHI), and the American Council on Science and Health (ACSH). I've used many of the resources of these organizations in preparing this book, and you can use these same resources to help decide if a proposed treatment is really appropriate for you.

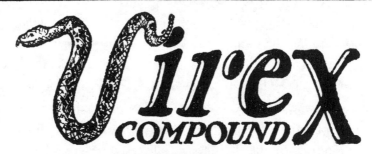

COURTESY OF THE AMA ARCHIVES

Virex Compound, distributed by Dale Laboratories in Kansas City, Missouri.

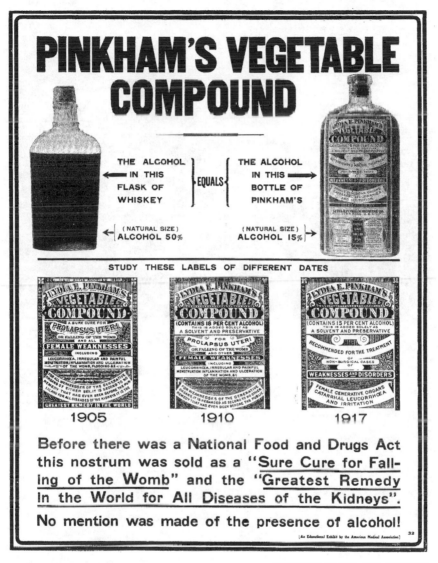

PINKHAM'S VEGETABLE COMPOUND

THE ALCOHOL IN THIS FLASK OF WHISKEY } EQUALS { THE ALCOHOL IN THIS BOTTLE OF PINKHAM'S

(NATURAL SIZE) ALCOHOL 50%

(NATURAL SIZE) ALCOHOL 15%

STUDY THESE LABELS OF DIFFERENT DATES

1905   1910   1917

Before there was a National Food and Drugs Act this nostrum was sold as a "Sure Cure for Falling of the Womb" and the "Greatest Remedy in the World for All Diseases of the Kidneys".

No mention was made of the presence of alcohol!

[An Educational Exhibit by the American Medical Association]

COURTESY OF THE AMA ARCHIVES

One of the most popular remedies of her time was Lydia Pinkham's Vegetable Compound for "female complaints and weaknesses," which featured Lydia's smiling face. She was the best-known female face in America when she died in 1883; at the time, her compound brought in about $300,000 a year, with over half spent on advertising. The company was family run until 1968 and the compound was still made (in Puerto Rico) in the late 1980s.

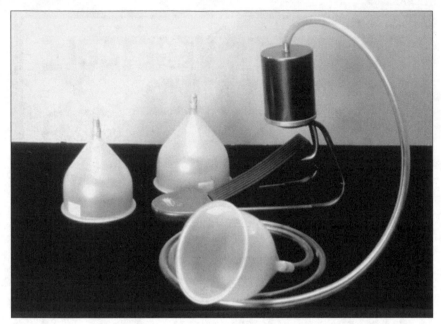

COURTESY OF BOB MCCOY AND THE MUSEUM OF QUESTIONABLE MEDICAL DEVICES

Foot-operated breast enlarger in three sizes. It produced a strong suction when operated, but any changes (including bruises and discomfort) were only temporary. In 1976 four million women responded to an ad selling this device for $9.95 plus postage.

chapter 3

Managed Care— The Biggest MediScam of All?

Putting a Price on Human Lives

"**YOUR MOTHER MIGHT NOT** make it," the doctor told us.

My older brother Bill and I, my two sisters, plus several nephews and nieces had taken over one of those haphazard waiting areas that every hospital has scattered among the various ERs and specialty care units. The attempt to create a living-room like atmosphere with lavender sofas and table lamps could not disguise the glare from the nurses' stations, the screech of the intercoms, or that nauseating antiseptic smell.

We were angry. None of us looked at the doctor, and none of us spoke. Our eyes and throats were too dry from crying, yelling, and not enough sleep. My mother might not make it, this doctor had said. How did he know any better than all the other doctors? Just a day earlier, some other specialist had reported that my mother had recovered and was doing fine—again.

The doctor was standing, rocking on his heels and staring at his clipboard. "If she's not kept on life support, she's going to die," he said.

Finally someone was telling us the truth. Finally, we could decide for ourselves—and for her. "There'll be no life support for me," she'd always said. She'd even written it into her will.

I begin this chapter with a personal story of health care crime, one that illustrates the pitfalls of managed care, including health maintenance organizations (HMOs), preferred provider organizations (PPOs), independent physician associations (IPAs), and the whole alphabet soup of similar organizations lumped under the banner of "managed care." This story wasn't part of one of my undercover investigations. This was real life—*my* real life, as well as that of my family. And in this story I learned lessons the hard way, enduring firsthand the resulting tragedy.

What can you learn from these experiences? That the treatment you receive from an HMO doctor or hospital is only as good as your HMO, because that organization tells your doctor and hospital what they can and cannot do.

My mother, Helen Whitlock, was an honest, hard-working woman of inspiring stamina and guts. And it took her HMO little more than a week to destroy all that. Her HMO (and the managed-care system in general) is responsible, my family believes, for putting her on a horrific roller-coaster ride of misdiagnoses and mistreatment which hastened her death.

My mother raised me and my three brothers and two sisters all by herself. We all called her "Ma." When I was young, she had dark brown hair and piercing blue eyes. She seemed so mighty then, though she was a small woman—five foot one, 110 pounds. A survivor of the Great Depression, she'd worked at Appleton Electric Company in Chicago all her adult life. Having attended college, she started out as a secretary. But Ma saw no reason why she couldn't transfer out to the shop and run the machinery. After all, the pay was better.

She was tough enough to take on what was traditionally a man's job. Once, her hair got caught in a machine and a lot of it was torn out. She kept on working. Another time, a machine bore a screw deep into her hand. The doctor had to resort to a screwdriver to extract the screw. She kept on working.

"She never complained about nuthin'," as my brother Bill says. Whenever she was sick, she went in the bedroom and came back out again when she was well. Later in life, she fought emphysema for ten years.

She was still tough at eighty-two years of age, relatively healthy and full of energy. She still had those piercing blue eyes. She'd moved to Las

Alamedas, California, and bought a condominium near Bill and my sister Alice. They went out to dinner two or three times a week. She played cards.

Then Ma started feeling more and more tired. She started going to a general practitioner who worked for her HMO out of a clinic in nearby Long Beach. The doctor said only that she was taking her medication incorrectly. She didn't need to see a specialist, he insisted; besides, the HMO wouldn't allow it. Still, her problem continued for two or three months.

On a splendid Southern California Friday, in the late afternoon, Ma had problems breathing. Her blood pressure fell. "I'm feeling bad," she said. She'd never said that before.

My brother and sister tried calling Ma's doctor but couldn't reach him. They took her to the ER at a local hospital. She had low blood pressure, a doctor said, and her kidneys weren't working properly. Bill and Alice tried her doctor again—to get copies of her medical records. Their efforts to reach him were pointless, as it turned out. Ma's HMO told them that, since they'd brought her to the ER, they had in effect switched doctors. Ma's old doctor was not her doctor anymore. Period. HMOs save us money that way.

It was now late Friday evening. The HMO had not authorized the hospital to run extensive (meaning expensive) tests on Ma, so the hospital had her stay the night. The next day she was assigned a new doctor, a cardiologist, who did little more than accuse Bill and Alice of leaving Ma alone too much. "Nonsense!" said Bill. "We take her out to dinner, we play cards together and that's just for starters."

"You should put her in a nursing home," insisted the cardiologist.

Saturday afternoon. Another doctor arrived, this one a specialist in antibiotics. Tests showed that Ma had an infected heart valve. This doctor planned to insert a tube up her arm and into her heart, to drip antibiotics directly onto her valves. But without her medical records, he said she'd have to wait for more tests because he didn't know anything about Ma's drug and allergy history. Meanwhile she took antibiotics orally.

Bill and Alice waited until Monday; by this time, Ma was on oxygen. They couldn't get her to eat, and she was sleeping a lot. She could talk, though, and still showed her spunk. She pulled out her intravenous needle just to show them she could.

The hospital physician, on instructions from the HMO, ignored Ma's old doctor. No one seemed to care about getting her records. Still, Bill and Alice were able to contact the doctor. "I can't do anything," he told them matter-of-factly (he'd obviously been through this before). "I'm not her doctor anymore." His hands, it seems, were tied.

The tube to the heart was finally scheduled to go in on Thursday, almost a week after my brother and sister had brought Ma in. Once the tube was in, the doctors told them, they'd have to move Ma to a nearby nursing home. Bill and Alice objected. Ma would be too fragile, they explained, and she'd have a tube running up her arm and into her heart. Bill pleaded with the doctors, who couldn't help since their orders had come from the HMO. Bill appealed to the HMO. It refused to budge.

The tube was inserted, the antibiotic delivered, and later that day an ambulance took Ma to the nursing home. She was conscious and seemed to be doing all right, so they left to let her sleep.

Within three hours, my brother Bill returned to the home to find Ma unconscious and alone. The tube up her arm was gone. Bill became unglued and screamed at the nurse who had pulled the tube. No one, not even she, could say why. The nurse was just following orders. It had become a farce, like one of those dark comedies that portray hospitals as death traps staffed by bumbling incompetents. Trembling, Bill called the HMO.

"I need to talk to somebody," he told them, "because they're killing my mother! They're killing her!"

Only then did her HMO throw Ma a bone. It approved her trip back to the hospital. We all wondered how much of this moving around Ma could take. To her, it must have felt like a beating. How could it not? Her kidneys were failing, and she'd developed pneumonia caused by low blood pressure.

By that time, concerned family members started to gather.

Back to the hospital. The next day, a Saturday (at least, I think it was a Saturday—no one was sleeping much at the time), there was yet another specialist to reinsert the tube into her heart. That afternoon, everyone went home for a brief time. We returned to a crisis. Ma was gasping for breath as the nurses scrambled to give her oxygen. Ma was biting at them and screaming, "I can't breathe! I can't breathe when they put that oxygen on!"

Bill said something like, "She's dying right here in their hands."

He wasn't far from the truth. Ma was suffering from congestive heart failure (CHF), which meant that excess fluid was accumulating around her heart and lungs. The oxygen they were giving her made her lungs expand, which caused them to press against her heart—leaving the blood and other fluids nowhere to go. Any nurse should have known that giving oxygen is the last thing you should be doing for a patient with CHF and emphysema. But they *didn't know* she had CHF or emphysema. Alice had to remind them of that and anything else she could think of, again and again and with every new doctor.

"Don't any of you read the patient's charts?" Alice asked. They only shrugged.

They "saved" Ma just in time. They moved Ma to the intensive-care unit, where she was able to sleep. The doctors told us she was doing much better. So did she. "I'm doing better, I am," she said. But those blue eyes of hers had lost their glimmer. The family could tell she'd all but given up.

Two more days passed. I thought and hoped that the worst of the nightmare was over. But the next day Ma was back in the ER—on life support. Bill and Alice arrived to find doctors and nurses scrambling. They were shouting, pushing everyone out of the way.

And that brings us back to the waiting room where I began this chapter. In the end it was peaceful. They unplugged her, and she went fast. On January 30, 1997, she died of heart failure due to infected valves of the heart.

When he finally left her bed, Bill muttered to one of the nurses, "I guess you did your best."

The nurse stopped and stared. Her face was ashen and blank, her eyes glossy. "Oh, no, we didn't," she muttered back.

"The HMO tried to save a few bucks and Ma's dead as a result," Bill said later. "They kill by neglect, and they don't care if it's your mother or their dad."

Two months later, as the pain was just starting to fade, Ma's old doctor called Bill. He wanted to know how Ma was doing.

FALLING BETWEEN THE CRACKS IN MANAGED CARE

I hope my story doesn't sound familiar to your family, though I wouldn't be surprised if it does. A recent report by the Institute of Medicine estimated that at least 44,000 and perhaps as many as 98,000 hospitalized Americans die every year from medical mistakes.

How many of these mistakes are exacerbated by the managed-care system? A good many, to be sure. One 1998 poll showed that almost 50 percent of Americans reported they or someone they know has had problems getting necessary care from an HMO—things like being refused access to a specialist, difficulties in getting their HMO to cover an emergency-room bill, or having to go through an appeals process because care was denied.

Sadly, Ma's tale is only one of too many. Consider what happened to James X. Lightfoote (not his real name). According to Carol Eisenberg in a *Newsday* article, back in February of 1998, Lightfoote, a forty-five-year-old letter carrier, was seriously considering suicide. It wasn't his rare and deadly bile duct cancer that had driven him to such desperation. It was his HMO.

On February 19, the day before he was scheduled to undergo surgery at a Manhattan hospital, Lightfoote's wife got a phone call from a hospital official. Could they come up with $52,000 by 2:30 P.M.? If not, the surgery could not be performed.

To the Lightfootes, it felt like extortion, like something out of a Mafia movie. How could they possibly come up with so much money in such little time?

Frantic, his wife dug out every credit card she could find. But they couldn't come up with the money.

James, listening in, began to plan suicide.

How did the Lightfootes end up in such a predicament? It had been little over a month since his doctor diagnosed the cancer. The doctor had told him that the tumor was spreading rapidly and would soon be inoperable. What's more, the surgery itself would be complicated. His life depended on finding a capable surgical specialist—immediately.

Lightfoote and his wife had requested referral to such a specialist, but their HMO snubbed them at every turn. No surgeon on the plan's specialty referral list could do such work. Worse, the HMO would not pay for a doctor outside its plan. Finally the HMO referred the Lightfootes to a cancer surgeon on its list. The HMO considered him qualified to operate on Lightfoote—but was he? Other surgeons said that the man had had little experience with bile duct cancer.

Meanwhile the cancer was eating away at James Lightfoote's insides.

Lightfoote found it easier to fight the cancer than his managed-care provider. Just finding a way through the maze of the HMO's guidelines was a full-time job. It became clear to Peggy Lightfoote that the only way to save her husband's life was by borrowing money and refinancing their home.

Two friends withdrew money from their retirement savings, giving the Lightfootes checks totaling $45,000. Then the Lightfootes remortgaged their house to pay the first installment for the surgery. March came, and James was still alive. The surgery was rescheduled, and the operation was successful.

James Lightfoote regrets the day he decided to ditch his old fee-for-service plan for an HMO. He'd hoped to save a few bucks. Instead the HMO gave him one chilling rejection after another that nearly cost him his life.

In the last decade, tens of millions of people like my mother and James Lightfoote have moved from fee-for-service insurance into managed care—and many are denied care, just when they need their insurance most. Hopefully my stories will make you better prepared, if not outraged. Because, believe it or not, James Lightfoote's tale may be one of the happier ones.

FAILING TO MEET TREATMENT CRITERIA

David Goodrich, a deputy district attorney in San Bernardino, California, battled a rare form of stomach cancer for three years before dying in 1995. For two of those grueling years, his HMO delayed and denied approval for the experimental high-dose chemotherapy treatments recommended by his doctors. The plan insisted that Goodrich was not "an appropriate candidate" for this therapy because his cancer had progressed too far.

The HMO conceded that none of the network doctors had the knowledge to treat Goodrich's rare cancer. Like James Lightfoote, David Goodrich needed a specialist. Like Lightfoote, Goodrich faced dead end after dead end. Finally he sought treatment outside his managed-care plan—but without first getting the plan's approval. Because of that, the HMO refused to pay. By then, though, it was too late anyway.

FINANCIAL INCENTIVES TO NOT TREAT

Like any insurance company, HMOs and other managed-care plans profit by taking in more money in premiums than they pay out in claims. But unlike traditional medical insurance, where doctors and hospitals are paid for providing their patients with medical services, HMO doctors and hospitals make money by *not* providing services. The concept is called "risk-sharing."

In traditional medical insurance, your insurer carries all of the financial risks. Your doctor and hospital provide whatever services they think appropriate and the insurance company pays the bill, minus your deductible. If you were to receive, say, a surgery you really didn't need, only you and your insurance company would suffer. Your doctor and hospital would both profit financially.

In HMOs and many other managed-care plans, doctors and hospitals are paid a flat fee for every patient enrolled in their care, whether the patient is actually seen or not. Although these payments are sharply discounted from normal fee-for-service charges, they are predictable and reliable sources of income. And they represent risk-sharing because, in return for those fixed but reliable payments, the doctors and hospitals now assume the financial burden of providing the patient with all appropriate medical care. Under this system, should you receive an unnecessary operation, the doctor and hospital pay for it out of their own pockets. The flip side of this arrangement is that, if you *didn't* get an operation you really *did* need, the doctor and hospital would pocket the savings under some plans. And that's exactly what happens sometimes.

Take the case of Patrick Shea, a computer executive from Minnesota. He was experiencing shortness of breath and dizzy spells, and had a family history of heart problems. He wanted to see a cardiologist. But his HMO doctor assured him there was no need to see a specialist.

Shea suffered more chest pains during a trip overseas and had to be hospitalized there. Again his doctor told him a specialist was not necessary. His problems were stress-related, the doctor maintained.

Shea never did see a specialist. He died of a heart attack at the age of forty in March 1993, leaving his wife with two young children and troubling questions. An autopsy disclosed that he had suffered from arteriosclerosis—blocked arteries in his heart—which probably could have been corrected with cardiac bypass surgery.

Hospitals, too, benefit by minimizing the number of services provided to HMO patients. Imagine you owned an apartment building where one thousand people paid their rent every month but never actually lived there. No upkeep, no maintenance, no wear and tear on the infrastructure, and minimal utility bills. In a profit-making, freestanding hospital, the goal is to fill 100 percent of the beds because the hospital makes money by delivering services. But in an HMO hospital, the goal is zero-percent occupancy—because they make their money by *not* delivering services.

And we, as patients, are stuck in the middle. On the one hand, traditional medical insurance offers doctors and hospitals incentives to offer us medical services we don't need, while managed care offers incentives to deny us medical services we *do* need. Your best bet is to find a conscientious, ethical physician who places his or her patients' needs above every other consideration, and is willing to fight the HMO or other payer to make sure that the patient receives all necessary medical care.

THE PERVASIVENESS OF MANAGED CARE

Eighty to eighty-five percent of all Americans who have health care insurance are covered by managed-care plans. According to an article by Christine Gorman for *Time* it's estimated that managed care saved from $150 billion to $250 billion in 1997 alone. But in exchange for the stable premiums sought by employers, those insured by managed care have given up the freedom to see any doctor or specialist anytime they want unless they are willing to pay more. Despite popular belief, consumers are not the only ones making sacrifices. Managed-care plans pinch doctors' incomes and also review the doctors' treatment plans, sometimes overruling them. This is the infamous "pre-certification" process. Hospitals and drug companies, too, are forced to shave profit margins in order to land managed-care contracts.

Likewise, other health care institutions and industries also share conflicting goals. The government, through Medicare and Medicaid, hurts patients by underpaying for most services. Doctors and hospitals make up for this by overcharging patients who have private insurance, which drives up our insurance premiums. And the HMOs are hurting us by limiting or denying physician and hospital services, diagnostic tests, and treatments. If that weren't enough, the government, HMOs and, yes, even insurance companies have a new trick up their sleeves—fixed payments. Together, the payers inform the health care providers that they will only pay a fixed amount for a particular service, without regard to how much it costs to provide that particular service. So, if it costs a provider of health care services $5,000 to do a first-class job of removing your gall bladder but your insurance company will only pay $3,000, guess what might happen?

Cutbacks. Compromises. Shorter surgery time. Less anesthesia. One less operating nurse to take care of you. Transfer to an outpatient surgical center without an overnight stay. In short, the quality of your care drops—possibly to dangerous levels. And all the while, the HMO dictates your health care with an iron hand.

CUTTING CARE TO CUT COSTS

Gorman's article on managed care in *Time* cites many HMO horror stories. One woman's new daughter, Joan (not her real name), was born with a hole in her heart. Realizing that Joan might eventually need surgery, and considering the family's existing medical insurance to be inadequate, Joan's mother went looking for an HMO plan. Most plans considered Joan's condition to be "pre-existing," and therefore not covered. The mother was delighted when her insurance agent told her about a local HMO that would cover Joan, and switched to the plan.

When doctors determined that Joan did indeed need surgery two months later, her HMO declared a two-year minimum waiting period for coverage of pre-existing conditions. Now it would not pay for the surgery. Dead end.

Joan did receive the care she needed, no thanks to the HMO. In the end, a special state program for the poor paid the bill.

In 1994 a fifty-five-year-old woman discovered her body was terribly bruised following a trip to Honolulu from her home in Chicago. The diagnosis: aplastic anemia. She was told she needed a bone-marrow transplant immediately. Her son was a good match and was ready to fly to Hawaii to be the donor. Her HMO insisted that she fly back at her own expense to be treated in Chicago. If she declined, she would be refusing services. They wouldn't pay her bills if she was treated in Hawaii. Feeling she had no choice, the woman boarded a flight to the mainland where she suffered a stroke midflight. Nine days later, she died. The HMO disputed their client's account of the events, claiming that she had noticed brusing prior to her trip and should have seen a doctor then.

WHAT ARE WE PAYING HMO PREMIUMS FOR, ANYWAY?

We have a health care crisis on our hands. Our needs are great, but everyone's hands are tied, it seems.

There are few things worse than being denied coverage by your insurer in a time of dire need. You feel disappointed, betrayed, and abandoned. You paid for that coverage! If you didn't have insurance at all, then you'd expect to be out on your own. Now you're not only on your own, but the insurance company still has all that money you paid them to take care of you. In the end, you cope any way you can. Some of us deny ourselves further health care. Some try to heal themselves, others seek out the MediScammers, and a few commit suicide in total despair. Some fight the system and find that in many jurisdictions they cannot sue their HMO for damages. Others discover too late that a procedure, had it been given earlier, might have saved their lives.

HMO executives say their industry has been unfairly stigmatized by highly publicized horror stories. They point to widespread consumer satisfaction and a positive track record overall. Besides, they stress, the HMOs have helped stabilize once soaring health care costs.

But what does the public say? According to a 1999 Health Confidence Survey sponsored by the Employee Benefit Research Institute, the Consumer Health Education Council, and Matthew Greenwald and Associates, Inc., one-half of all Americans with health insurance were extremely or very satisfied with their current health insurance plan. Other findings:

- Respondents enrolled in fee-for-service plans are most likely to be satisfied with various aspects of the health care they've received over the past two years, while those in HMOs are least likely to be satisfied, even when it comes to areas considered to be the strength of HMOs, such as paperwork and costs.
- The same survey found that the people who were less satisfied and less confident about their health care system are those in managed care; those in poorer health; and women (considered to be the primary household decision makers with respect to family health care).

- Yet the survey unearthed that there's a tremendous amount of confusion about what managed care is and whether or not individuals are enrolled in it. Less than 20 percent responding felt very familiar with managed-care plans. And 54 percent of those surveyed based their opinions about managed care on what others have told them.
- Respondents enrolled in managed-care plans—whether or not they were aware of being in managed care—tend to be less satisfied with and less confident in the health care system than those in fee-for-service plans. This tendency is more pronounced among those experiencing greater degrees of managed care: respondents in HMOs are less likely to be satisfied or confident than those in PPO plans.
- Despite the proliferation of lower-cost alternatives to fee-for-service private insurance, the current cost of health insurance appears to be the primary reason respondents are uninsured.

HMO executives insist that many complaints result from consumers' misunderstandings. Indeed, the consumer makes an agreement when signing up with an HMO: In exchange for almost universally lower premiums, guaranteed renewability, and no lifetime or annual caps on coverage, you have to give up one thing—the right to go anywhere to get any treatment. Just stay within the plan and you'll be taken care of.

That old game again: It's *us*. We got it wrong. We should be thankful. But then, what if your HMO doesn't happen to provide the treatment you need? You'd better just hope you live long enough to wind your way through the bureaucracy as your HMO plots the least expensive pathway to coping with your problem.

In spite of what they tell us, HMOs' negligence persists. The stories are out there. So why can't we have a little say in our health care, or even protect ourselves?

The for-profit, managed-care industry must be held accountable. Patients like my mother and the Lightfootes should have the right to appeal denials of care to an impartial panel. As it stands, most appeals can only be made to the insurance carrier itself, and not to an outside party with the power to overrule the insurer's objections and compel it to pay for a necessary treatment. Patients should also have greater access to specialists and emergency care, and the freedom to sue companies if the patient suffers injury as a result of plan decisions. Currently, patients can sue doctors for malpractice, but federal law makes it difficult to sue a health insurer for coverage decisions.

ERISA—The Magic Shield for Managed Care

Marcia Frappert (not her real name) had leukemia and needed a bone-marrow transplant but her HMO refused to pay. The Frapperts appealed for months—they'd understood the transplant was supposed to be covered. The HMO finally reversed its decision, but it was too late to do Marcia any good. At age forty-six, she succumbed to the illness.

Her husband Zacariah (not his real name) decided to sue their HMO for wrongful death, but soon he learned that he could not sue an HMO in state court because of the 1974 federal Employee Retirement Income Security Act (ERISA). Even if Frappert had been successful in suing the plan in federal court, he could not have recovered punitive damages or compensation for all of his wife's pain and suffering. The only thing he would have been compensated for was the value of the care that was denied. But how do you compensate for the care that could have saved a life?

ERISA was enacted to address concerns about the mismanagement of private pension plans and to protect the interests of participants in their employee benefits plans. It's a little-known but all-pervasive law that effectively shields most health insurers from financial liability for their decisions to deny or limit coverage. While ERISA aimed at dealing with irregularities in large pension plans, its effect has been to shield insurance companies from "bad faith" lawsuits. And while the law does guarantee the insured various rights, trial by jury is not one of them. It creates no incentive for insurers to treat claims fairly. Frappert believes that insurance companies are using the law to avoid paying for treatments. Chances are,

ERISA applies to your own plan. It's believed that at least 125 million Americans are covered by employer-sponsored health plans that are sheltered by ERISA.

THE FALTERING PUSH FOR REFORM

Unfortunately, the federal law has not yet changed. But justice may be still be possible thanks to some state lawsuits. In 1996, the widow of David Goodrich, Teresa, sued Aetna Healthplans of California for its refusal to pay for high-dose chemotherapy which had been recommended by the HMO's own doctors for her husband; her suit alleged breach of contract and wrongful death due to the unreasonable conduct of the defendant.

In January 1999 a jury awarded her $116 million in punitive damages. By a 10–2 vote, the jury found that Aetna had committed "malice, oppression, and fraud" which had contributed to the shortening of the life of her husband, David Goodrich. This ruling came a week after the same jury had found Aetna liable for more than $4.5 million in compensatory damages for Goodrich's death. Aetna appealed, but the appellate court let stand the $120.5 million judgment.

Maybe the lawsuits are helping, or maybe it's plain old economics (my guess is the latter), but some HMOs are trying to change the way they do business. UnitedHealthcare's landmark decision to give doctors the final say on treatment decisions does seem revolutionary. Still, true reform, if it's to come, remains a long way off.

And if you think politicians can help, think again. Many states have tackled HMO issues, spawning a hodgepodge of inconsistent regulations. Yet state consumer protections don't help all those Americans with health plans exempt from state regulation.

On a positive note, Wisconsin recently joined more than a dozen states that have created independent review panels to hear appeals from people denied coverage by their insurance companies. The Wisconsin review panels, which are required to make their decisions within thirty days, have the authority to make insurers pay for certain treatments.

Meanwhile, in the U.S. Congress, the long-simmering question of how to regulate managed care continues. Republicans and Democrats in the Senate have drafted rival versions of a "Patients' Bill of Rights." Both sides address the most important issues, such as coverage of emergency room visits, access to medical specialists, and the right to an independent review when an HMO refuses to pay. As usual, party politics have gotten in the way of finding solutions. Republicans would defer to the states over the question of the rights of patients in HMOs. Democrats want more aggressive (which often means costlier) measures to limit the power HMOs have over the decisions made by doctors.

When it comes to lawsuits, the two parties part company. Generally speaking, Senate Democrats stand with physicians, personal-injury lawyers, and consumer groups, while Republicans have taken up the cause of employers and the managed-care industry. Taking the position that HMOs, like any other businesses, should be held legally accountable for their actions, Democrats argue against Republicans who claim that eliminating ERISA's protections would bring on a deluge of lawsuits. They fear that omitting the ERISA umbrella would send premiums sky-high. Higher premiums could result in a decline in employer-provided health care benefits.

I side with the Democrats on this issue: The threat of damages could deter HMOs from denying legitimate patient care once and for all. Accountability could forever change the way HMOs do business—as well it should. Suppose, for example, that a police officer was only accountable for providing public safety, but allowed to do it in whatever way he or she saw fit. No further responsibilities. No liability or accountability for job performance. No need to respect the public's civil rights. What kind of law enforcement would we have?

Will a Patient's Bill of Rights be enacted anytime soon? Don't place any bets on it. Meanwhile, disenchanted patients continue to fight—and usually lose—the bitter battles over what managed-care organizations are obligated to pay for. In the months following the death of her husband, Dianne Shea, like Teresa Goodrich, sought to discover how her husband could have died of an undiagnosed disease. What she found outraged her. In her wrongful-death lawsuit, she claimed that her husband's doctor had an undisclosed financial conflict of interest in refusing to refer the patient to a cardiologist: She believes that her husband's doctor received extra compensation from their HMO for not sending patients to specialists. The defendants all denied any conflict of interest, as well as denying negligence in treating Shea. But Dianne Shea remains convinced that the cost-containment philosophy of managed care caused her husband's death.

But the case of Cynthia Herdrich did reach the Supreme Court. After Herdrich's physician required Herdrich to wait eight days for an ultrasound at an HMO facililty, her appendix ruptured, causing Herdrich peritonitis. Though she won a malpractice lawsuit against the doctor, she decided to sue the HMO, too.

In a unanimous decision, in June 2000 the U.S. Supreme Court handed down a ruling that HMOs couldn't be sued in federal court for rewarding doctors who contain costs by rationing patient treatment. The court stated that health care is traditionally subject to state regulation. Though HMOs claimed a decisive victory for the managed-care industry, others believe that the decision may open the floodgates for lawsuits at the state level.

SURVIVING THE MANAGED-CARE JUGGERNAUT

Regardless of the human costs, managed care does save money and is therefore cheaper than standard medical insurance. So, like it or not, most of us wind up resorting to a managed-care plan of some sort. Now what? How can we protect ourselves from having our health sacrificed in the name of corporate profits? How do we go about sizing up that lumbering, faceless managed-care company that's based in some obscure suburb many of its subscribers have never heard of? Here are a few tips:

- Remember that there are many managed-care plans out there to choose from. And don't be suckered into thinking that the one with the lowest monthly payment will always have the lowest total costs for health care. Look at co-payments, deductibles, and noncovered services. What preventative services do they cover? What about emergency care? Make sure that you understand what the plan *doesn't* cover.

- Keep in mind that managed-care plan representatives are trying to sell you something. They make money by convincing you that their particular health plan is the best one for you. As the old song goes, "It ain't necessarily so!" Shop for health care coverage with the same wary skepticism that you use when shopping for a car or house.

- Make sure that you read all the plan's literature. Read a copy of the contract, and make sure you understand all the limitations and exclusions that are conditions of service. Make sure you understand what services are included in your coverage, and which are not. If there is anything you don't understand, ask the sales representative to explain it to you. Then ask to have the explanation written out in plain, simple English. Some sales reps will *tell* you whatever it takes to get you to sign the contract. But when it comes to putting their promises down on paper, you may see them suddenly start to backpedal.

- Check out the plan's provider directory. Is there a wide selection of primary-care providers? This choice is critical, because you'll need someone in your corner who's willing to go to bat for your health care needs. Are there major hospitals in your area? How close are the medical facilities to where you will receive routine and emergency care? Do they have a wide variety of specialists that you can be referred to?

- Ask people who belong to the plan if they're satisfied with the service they receive. What problems have they experienced?

- To avoid a shock, know your rights. Ask in advance for a list of drugs and conditions your plan doesn't cover. Can you, at any time, switch primary-care providers within the network? If so, there are likely to be conditions. Find out what they are. Since specialized care costs more, HMOs tend to limit access to such services. The primary-care physician determines whether or not a member needs to see a specialist, and then makes the appropriate referral. Ask for a copy of the contract the plan offers participating physicians, then read it to learn what the doctor's incentives may be to *not* refer you to a specialist.

- Look for a plan that covers all of your specific and anticipated health needs—mammograms if you're a woman over age forty, chronic conditions if you have an asthmatic child, and alternative therapies such as chiropractic, if that's what you prefer. Does the plan you're considering offer a wide range of preventive services? In the long run, preventive services can be the most cost-effective way to stay healthy.
- Once you've signed, don't accept unsatisfactory care. Become the squeaking wheel that gets the grease. If you're not happy with your treatment, follow the grievance procedures outlined in your contract exactly. Ask your primary-care provider to help, and tell your employee-benefits coordinator at work to contact the managed-care provider personally.

chapter 4

Dangerous Doctors

Physicians Are Supposed to Police Each Other—
Why Don't They Do a Better Job of It?

IN 1985 JEROME Z. COUGAR (not his real name), forty-four, was living a pleasant, upper-middle-class lifestyle in suburban Fort Worth, Texas. His position as a cost estimator for a defense contractor afforded him a comfortable living and allowed his wife to stay home with their three children. About the only significant problem in his life was chronic lower back pain. He had no way of knowing that his search for relief of that pain was about to tear his life apart.

Tests revealed that Cougar's back problems were caused by a herniated L5-S1 vertebral disc. In other words, the pad of cartilage that separated the lowest part of his backbone from his pelvis was bulging inward and pinching the spinal cord. Cougar's orthopedic surgeon recommended surgery to remove the disc and fuse the two bones together. That would permanently remove the pressure on Cougar's spinal cord and, it was expected, eventually result in a complete recovery.

Like the vast majority of patients, Cougar was not involved in selecting the anesthesiologist who would care for him during surgery. That choice was left to his surgeon, and he chose Garry E. Winn, a former chief of anesthesiology at the hospital.

The choice of an anesthesiologist is not to be taken lightly. Anesthesiologists do more than just keep the patient out of pain. They must monitor the patient constantly during surgery for signs that something is amiss. They are responsible for the single most important factor in any surgical procedure—making sure that the patient's brain is receiving enough oxygen. If the supply of oxygenated blood to the brain is interrupted, brain cells begin dying in less than five minutes.

Winn had been unusually busy that April, handling over one hundred anesthesia cases—about twice his usual patient load. The previous month, Winn's two former partners, anesthesiologists Gary L. Neisler and Kenneth C. Ponitz, had forced Winn out of their group, and surgeon sympathy for Winn was running high. The surgeons might have been less eager to work with Winn had they known he'd been ousted because two patients in his care had recently died under circumstances that gave rise to grave concerns about his competency.

Winn's personal history contained a number of incidents that suggested he might have been impaired physically or intellectually. In 1982, while being treated for bleeding of the stomach, he suffered a stroke that produced right-side weakness and difficulty in speaking. After several months of physical therapy, Winn returned to his anesthesia practice, telling his colleagues he'd recovered 95 percent of his motor skills. But several surgeons reported to his partners Neisler and Ponitz that they would no longer work with Winn. Most said only that they weren't "comfortable" with him, but at least a few complained that Winn was becoming inattentive and indecisive during surgery.

In 1984 concern about Winn's mental deterioration led his partners to request that Winn be evaluated by a neurologist, a physician who specializes in disorders of the brain. Winn agreed, and flew to Columbia University in New York for the evaluation. There the neurologist discovered that the blood flow to Winn's brain was constricted enough to limit his reasoning abilities. It was recommended that Winn consider having surgery. Instead Winn flew home and told his partners that he'd been given a clean bill of health.

Winn was also a chronic alcoholic who, by his own admission, was consuming between one and two pints of vodka every day. On top of this, he was taking Atarax, a potent sedative normally used to relax patients before anesthesia. The AMA defines "impairment" as the "inability to practice medicine with reasonable skill and safety to patients" because of physical illness, alcoholism, or drug dependence. At the time of Jerome Z. Cougar's surgery, anesthesiologist Garry Winn was impaired in all three categories.

During one of the diagnostic tests performed prior to the surgery, Cougar had been found to be hypersensitive to the narcotic Demerol. This placed Cougar at a special risk for general anesthesia, since such patients tend to overreact to other narcotics as well. Therefore, Winn decided to use a spinal block, a procedure in which the patient is kept awake and the lower part of the body deadened with nonnarcotic drugs injected directly into the spinal column.

The surgery took place the following afternoon. For the first forty-five minutes, everything went as planned. Then Cougar complained of pain as the surgeon tugged on a nerve. In response, Winn injected Cougar with one and possibly two milliliters of Sufenta, a narcotic many times more potent than Demerol. Because Sufenta can cause even those with normal narcotic tolerance to stop breathing, the standard procedure at that point would have been for the anesthesiologist to intubate the patient, which involves inserting a breathing tube down the throat and into the lungs, then connecting this tube with a ventilator that breathes for the patient. Winn did not do this. At this critical moment in his patient's life, Winn became distracted by the surgery and forgot to monitor Cougar's breathing and heart rate.

About ten to twelve minutes later, a nurse alerted everyone that Cougar *wasn't* breathing and had turned blue. Winn hesitated, suggesting that they wait a few more minutes to "see what happens." The surgeon himself ordered the patient intubated and ventilated, then completed the operation.

In the recovery room Winn removed the breathing tube and ventilator. Even under normal circumstances, when a patient is removed from a ventilator, the standard procedure is to order a test of the blood gases to make sure that the patient's own breathing is providing enough oxygen and removing enough carbon dioxide to continue without the ventilator. Winn failed to do this, committing yet another major error.

The brain swells after it has been injured by oxygen deprivation, and elevated blood carbon dioxide makes the problem worse; for the brain, completely enclosed in the skull, this creates a situation similar to blowing up a balloon inside of a bottle. With no place to expand, the pressure inside the brain increases. This makes it even harder for the vitally needed oxygenated blood to get in, and the damage worsens. According to expert testimony at the subsequent malpractice trial, Cougar should have been kept on the ventilator until he was fully awake and his blood oxygen and carbon dioxide were normal.

That night Cougar began having seizures. Winn was called at home but, despite the clear emergency of the situation, didn't arrive for another hour and twenty minutes. He later explained that he'd fallen back asleep after the call. Winn reintubated Cougar and connected him to a ventilator. But the damage had already been done. Cougar's mental processes remained normal, but he was left severely speech-impaired, without bowel or bladder control, and with a seizure disorder. He was confined to a wheelchair.

The most terrifying aspect of this case is not that a brain-damaged, drug-abusing alcoholic was practicing medicine, but that he was surrounded by competent, non-impaired physicians who failed to stop him. Even after the Cougar incident, Winn was permitted to resign from practicing anesthesia at his hospital and instead go into general practice. Winn died in 1990, never having been formally disciplined by the medical community.

The Cougar family sued not only Winn but the hospital itself, along with all six anesthesiologists on its staff, plus the hospital's chief of staff. Winn himself declared bankruptcy before the trial began and didn't even bother to attend after jury selection.

At trial, no one contested that Winn's treatment of Cougar was grossly negligent. The only real issue was why they hadn't tried to stop Winn from treating patients in the first place.

In the end the jury found Winn liable for gross negligence. They also found Neisler, Ponitz, the hospital, and its chief of staff negligent for their failure to stop Winn, and assessed the defendants a total of $14 million in damages—$5 million to be paid by the doctors and the remainder to be paid by the hospital.

HOW PHYSICIANS ARE *SUPPOSED* TO BE DISCIPLINED

The medical profession is supposed to police its own ranks for the simple reason that, except in the most egregious of cases, it takes a competent physician to recognize an incompetent one. In theory, the medical community has established a multitiered system for weeding out bad doctors on the local, state, and national levels. Still, impaired, criminal, psychotic, and incompetent physicians often are allowed to continue harming patients for years before they are stopped—sometimes, they never are.

It's important to realize that the law itself places very few restrictions on a properly licensed physician's conduct. There's nothing in the law to prevent, say, a doctor from prescribing birth control pills to treat an earache or to prevent a family practitioner from practicing brain surgery in his office.

Instead of laws, the medical community evaluates practitioners by what are called "standards of care." These standards are set by physicians themselves and are necessarily flexible because medicine is as much art as science, requiring room for individual judgment. The critical issue is that the physician must exercise "reasonable care and skill" in delivering care. Suppose, for example, you see three physicians for the same infection. Dr. A prescribes an antibiotic that cures your infection quickly but has frequent side effects. Dr. B prescribes a different antibiotic that acts more slowly but causes fewer side effects. Dr. C prescribes an antibiotic that doesn't work at all on your type of infection and causes many side effects. Although Drs. A and B prescribed different antibiotics based on different judgments, both were practicing within the standard of care. Dr. C, on the other hand, is practicing below the standard of care because a reasonable physician would not have prescribed that drug for your condition. Standards of care also vary according to medical specialty and according to location. Thus, an obstetrician delivering babies in a major teaching hospital will be held to a higher standard of care than a family practitioner delivering babies in a remote rural hospital.

A number of agencies and professional associations are responsible for policing physicians to make sure that the standards of care are met; these include the following:

Hospitals

Physicians must apply for, and periodically renew, "privileges" at any hospital where they practice. These privileges specify what treatments or procedures the doctor is allowed to conduct in that hospital. To receive or renew privileges, the physician is supposed to present credentials or demonstrate personally that he or she has the training and skills to justify those privileges. The hospitals also have "peer review" committees of physicians and other professionals whose job is to review applications for privileges and to investigate complaints against the doctors on their staff.

On the hospital level, discipline can consist of limiting, suspending, or revoking a physician's privileges. If this happens, the hospital is usually obligated to report the action to the state medical board. But hospitals rarely revoke privileges, for two main reasons. The first is economic: Hospitals make money by having doctors admit and treat patients in their facilities. Revoking the privileges of someone like a heart surgeon could cost the hospital millions of dollars in revenue every year. The second reason is cronyism. The peer reviewers are colleagues and often friends of the physicians they are supposed to police. This often results in the attitude of, "Hey, I could be the one under investigation next time." As such, peer reviewers too often accept the denial of misconduct by a doctor over the repeated complaints of nurses and patients, dismissing their allegations out of hand.

Even when overwhelming evidence shows that a dangerous doctor is in their midst, peer reviewers often choose the easy way out and let the offender quietly resign from the hospital staff. This allows the dangerous doctor to simply transfer to another hospital, leaving no trail of his or her misdeeds.

State, County, and Local Medical Societies

Although these professional associations are supposed to work toward quality improvement in medical care, they often amount to little more than social clubs, and have no power to revoke or suspend medical licenses of their members—let alone those doctors who aren't members. While these societies can revoke an offending doctor's membership, this is a largely symbolic move since such membership is in no way required in order to practice medicine in the first place. Yet it is with local medical societies that most patient complaints about doctors are lodged. Usually the societies will have a mechanism for investigating complaints and mediating solutions between doctor and patient. Unresolved complaints can be forwarded to the state medical board, but this rarely happens, especially when the doctor in question is a member of the society.

State Medical Boards

These are the agencies responsible for licensing doctors. Their powers include the ability to revoke or suspend medical licenses. Disciplinary actions of this type become public information. The state boards also have milder forms of discipline that include probation and consent letters in which the physician agrees to abide by disciplinary conditions set down by the board in order to avoid harsher punishment. These actions usually don't become public.

How effective are the state medical boards? In 1999, there were 3,838 prejudicial actions taken by all state medical boards, according to the Federation of State Medical Boards. That's less than one-half of one percent of the nation's 797,600 licensed physicians. Even the medical boards admit that's not enough. The problem, they say, is that virtually no state medical board has the resources to investigate every complaint it receives. The Arizona Medical Board, for example, has only seven investigators to handle more than one thousand complaints a year.

Specialty Boards

Every recognized medical specialty has at least one professional board. These provide "board certification" for their members, showing that the doctors have met the criteria of professional competence necessary to become recognized specialists in their fields. Some specialty boards also require that members engage in continuing medical education activities in order to keep their membership current. The policing actions of specialty boards are limited to revoking the "board-certified" status of an errant member, and reporting him or her to the state medical board. Neither of these actions will, by itself, impair a doctor's ability to practice medicine.

National Practitioner Data Bank (NPDB)

Until recently, physicians who had their licenses yanked in one state could simply move across state lines and apply for another as was the case with Dr. Brown in chapter 1. The idea of the NPDB was to establish a single, unified database covering all disciplinary actions taken against all doctors nationwide. Even successful malpractice suits must be reported, including ones in which the doctor settles out of court. So far, the NPDB has disciplinary files on about 130,000 doctors and dentists.

The problem is that the information in the NPDB is only available to state medical boards, hospitals, HMOs, and organizations that employ doctors. The public is barred from obtaining the very information meant to protect it.

Public Citizen, the Washington, D.C.-based consumer advocacy organization, recently published *20,125 Questionable Doctors*. According to Public Citizen's August 8, 2000, press release about the book, the guide is the only publicly available national listing of doctors disciplined from 1990 through December 1999.

Public Citizen states that this country's system to protect its citizens from medical incompetence is inadequate. With a rate of serious disciplinary actions by state medical boards of only 3.5 per 1,000 doctors, the organization states that medical boards are way too lenient when disciplining doctors. The majority of doctors disciplined for the most serious offenses—sexual abuse or sexual misconduct, incompetence, negligence, substandard care, criminal conviction, overprescribing or misprescribing drugs, or substance abuse—weren't required to stop practicing even temporarily. Though 91 percent of all the disciplinary actions were for serious offenses, only 48 percent resulted in license probation, revocation, suspension, or surrender.

What does this mean to the patients of these doctors? The doctors are probably still practicing, and their patients probably know nothing about their offenses.

The unfortunate truth is that the medical community's "self-policing" of its own ranks stops very few errant physicians from practicing medicine. And when competent doctors fail in their duty to protect the public from rogue physicians, it is the criminal and civil justice systems that must step in and take over. Physicians argue, with justification, that malpractice suits are often unfair and drive up the cost of everyone's medical care. Yet, as the late attorney Melvin Belli was fond of pointing out, were it not for the rising cost of malpractice insurance and the threat of being sued for a colleague's errors, many doctors would be even less willing to help patrol their colleagues.

IMPAIRED PHYSICIANS

One of the largest classes of dangerous doctors, by far, is those impaired by drug and/or alcohol dependency. The problem is hardly new. Sigmund Freud, the founder of modern psychoanalysis, and William Halstead, the renowned nineteenth-century surgical pioneer, were both addicted to cocaine. But few patients—or physicians, for that matter—appreciate the true extent of the problem. According to a report by the AMA Council on Mental Health, of the known drug addicts in the United States and Europe, 15 percent are physicians and another 15 percent are in the nursing or pharmacy professions. In all, it is estimated that between 10 and 15 percent of all physicians in the U.S. are chemically dependent on drugs or alcohol or both.

It's important to keep in mind here that drug and alcohol abuse are not the only forms of physician impairment—just the only ones that the medical profession keeps track of. No one knows how many physicians are impaired by compulsive gambling, sexual disorders, head injury, stroke, Alzheimer's disease, or psychiatric disorders.

Why are there so many drug- and alcohol-abusing physicians? In part it's related to the tendency of physicians to have compulsive personalities that are naturally prone to addiction. In addition, physicians are subject to fatigue and stress from rigid schedules and excessively long working hours. Their knowledge of the workings of mood-altering drugs, plus their ready access to them, often results in their experimenting with drugs or alcohol as a means of dealing with stress.

The use of chemicals to relieve stress often begins in medical school, where alcohol and benzodiazepines—a drug family of sedatives that includes Valium—are the substances of choice. Older physicians, on the other hand, tend to prefer benzodiazepines and opiates—natural and synthetic drugs related to morphine—with family practitioners and anesthesiologists having the highest incidences of substance abuse.

Not surprisingly, the drugs of choice tend to vary among health care professions according to what is most readily available. Thus veterinarians are most likely to experiment with the animal anesthetic ketamine, dentists with nitrous oxide, nurses with painkillers, while pharmacists—who have ready access to most medications—tend to experiment with a mix of alcohol and small amounts of several different drugs. Anesthesiologists, who have unique access to the most potent drugs of all, tend to experiment with the extremely powerful and addictive class of narcotics that includes Sufenta.

While the FDA and Drug Enforcement Agency (DEA) require strict record-keeping by all those who dispense narcotics and other dangerous drugs, getting around the regulations is not difficult when the object is only to obtain enough drugs for personal consumption. An anesthesiologist, for example, can inject a patient with three milliliters of a drug, then write in the anesthesia record that he injected four milliliters and keep the difference. A nurse who is supposed to give a patient two pills can dispense one and pocket the other. A pharmacist can write off a certain amount of controlled substances as "wasted" or otherwise damaged in handling and discarded. Some physicians have even been convicted of "splitting" narcotics prescriptions with their patients, writing a prescription for, say, one hundred pills on condition that the patient return fifty to the doctor.

What Is Being Done?

Although the DEA and other federal agencies play an important part in identifying impaired physicians by reviewing prescription-drug records for "irregularities," it is again the medical community itself that is primarily responsible for policing its own ranks. While impaired physicians potentially face revocation or suspension of their medical licenses, as we have seen, this seldom happens. In cases where the physician is cooperative and making an apparently sincere effort to recover, the disciplinary action may be limited to a voluntary agreement to have his or her drug or alcohol usage monitored after release from a chemical-dependency treatment program.

Despite these options, the response of the medical community to the problem of impaired physicians is not encouraging. It is estimated that between one-third and one-half of all complaints about physicians to state medical boards involve allegations of substance abuse. Yet one study found that fewer than 5 percent of the documented disciplinary actions by one state medical board were related to emotional problems, including substance abuse. Nationwide, if we assume that only 10 percent of our physicians are chemically impaired, that is still around 79,760 doctors whose ability to practice medicine is being compromised by drugs or alcohol. Yet according to the Federation of State Medical Boards of the U.S., the oversight organization for the individual state medical boards, a total of only 607 physicians were formally disciplined for substance abuse in 1999. In other words, only 1 impaired physician in 100 faced action from his or her state medical board.

Although formal disciplinary actions taken by the state boards of medical examiners do become part of the public record, complaints received by them do not. Further, to encourage physicians to voluntarily come forward with their problems, most boards will authorize "private consent orders" in which the physician agrees to seek supervised treatment in lieu of formal disciplinary action. These private consent orders—and even the fact that a particular physician has signed one—are usually kept confidential. Likewise, actions taken by hospital peer review committees to deal with troublesome doctors also are kept confidential. For all these reasons, it is difficult to assess how diligent the medical community really is in rooting out impaired physicians. However, the mere fact that the percentage of impaired physicians is generally estimated to exceed 10 percent indicates that much more needs to be done.

The Patients Strike Back

If the medical profession itself is not doing enough to protect patients from impaired doctors, at least some courts are giving patients who are injured powerful weapons for striking back. One weapon, as shown by the Cougar case, allows patients to sue the impaired physician's hospital and colleagues on the allegation they should have recognized the obvious evidence that one of their own was impaired, then used the peer review process to discipline the offender. In some cases, malpractice plaintiffs list entire sections of the hospital medical staff as co-defendants on this allegation. It is hoped this threat will pressure competent physicians to pay closer attention to their colleagues' actions and alert the hospital's peer review committee when they suspect a fellow doctor is impaired or incompetent. Another weapon actually allows patients to sue the physician directly for not revealing his or her impaired status to them before treatment.

In 1994 William Z. Everet (not his real name), thirty-six, was examined by urologist Timothy S. Trulock of Albany, Georgia, for a lump on his penis. A urologist is a surgeon who specializes in treating problems of the urinary tract, including the genitals in males. Trulock diagnosed cancer of the penis without actually taking a tissue sample from the lump and having it examined to confirm the presence of cancer—the standard practice in such cases. Trulock convinced Everet to undergo surgery to remove the lump, assuring the patient that he would be back to work in a few days.

Shortly after the surgery, Everet began experiencing excruciating pain and a leftward bend in his penis during erection, which made sexual intercourse impossible. A visit with a different urologist revealed that Everet's true diagnosis was Peyronie's disease, an arthritis-like condition in which the tissues of the penis that cause erection become calcified. Peyronie's disease can be diagnosed by appropriate testing and is usually treated with vitamin E and medication instead of surgery. The condition generally goes away on its own over time.

Everet filed suit for malpractice, with his wife as co-plaintiff suing for loss of consortium. As the suit was being prepared for trial, Trulock was hospitalized after suffering a cocaine-induced seizure. He subsequently entered a substance abuse program. Because Trulock had self-reported his problems, the state's board of medical examiners entered into a private consent order with Trulock.

In pretrial testimony Trulock admitted to habitual cocaine use at about the time he had treated Everet. He also admitted that cocaine use could impair a physician's performance and judgment. But when specifically asked whether he had been under the influence of cocaine at the actual time he had treated Everet, Trulock refused to answer, citing his Fifth Amendment right against self-incrimination.

The principle allegations of Everet's suit were medical negligence, battery, and fraudulent concealment of Trulock's "illegal use and abuse of cocaine, substance abuse problem, and impairment." The battery claim was based on the legal theory that Everet would not have consented to surgery if he had known about Trulock's impairment; since battery is the unauthorized touching of another's person, Trulock allegedly committed battery by performing surgery on Everet under circumstances the patient had not authorized. The fraud claim was based on the theory that Trulock had held himself out to be a fully competent urologist when in fact he knew that he was not, by reason of chemical impairment.

At trial, the judge dismissed the battery claim and the jury found in favor of the urologist and the clinic on the medical-negligence claim. However, they found in favor of Everet and his wife on the claims for fraud and loss of consortium. The Everets were awarded $750,000 in damages plus $35,000 in punitive damages. Punitive damages are not generally covered by a physician's medical malpractice insurance and must be paid out of his or her own pocket. After some complicated legal maneuvering, the verdict was eventually upheld on appeal.

If an impaired physician commits fraud by holding him- or herself out as fully competent in a medical specialty, it logically follows that the patient's consent to treatment is not valid since it was obtained under fraudulent circumstances. That argument actually had been considered by an earlier court case.

In 1984 Paul X. O. Daniel (not his real name), fifty-nine, was examined by orthopedic surgeon Randall A. Williams of Metairie, Louisiana, for extreme degenerative back disease caused by spinal stenosis, a narrowing of the bones around the spinal cord. Williams recommended a decompressive laminectomy of the lower lumbar spine, an operation similar to but more extensive than the one Jerome Z. Cougar underwent. As a result of the surgery, Daniel was left without bowel or bladder control—a known, but rare, risk of the surgery.

Daniel initially sued Williams on the claim that Williams had not obtained informed consent because he did not properly educate the patient about the risks of surgery. Daniel had only a sixth-grade education and minimal reading skills, and had needed his wife's help to read the consent form, which listed the known risks of the surgery. He claimed that neither of them had understood that the listed risk of "loss of function of body organs" meant possible incontinence, and that he would not have consented to surgery had he been properly advised.

In 1986, Williams' medical license was suspended on grounds that included habitual alcohol abuse. Daniel then amended his claim to include the argument that he would not have consented to surgery had he known that Williams was a chronic alcoholic. Daniel died of unrelated causes before trial, and his widow proceeded to have the case tried before a judge, forgoing a jury trial. The judge agreed that Daniel had not given informed consent to surgery, both because Daniel had not been properly educated about his risks, and because Dr. Williams had not revealed his alcohol abuse. Daniel's widow was awarded $300,000. Although Williams appealed, the appellate court upheld the decision on the argument that patients have a right to know if their doctor is impaired, and that informed consent is not valid if the physician fails to disclose this fact before treatment.

The critical element in an informed-consent case is the assumption of risk. The theory behind obtaining informed consent is that a competent adult who has been properly educated and informed is able to assume the risks—legal as well as medical—of the treatment in question. This means the patient has little chance of recovering damages if he or she actually suffers one of those risks. In the absence of informed consent, however, it is the physician and hospital who bear those risks. That means that the patient who has not given informed consent may be able to recover damages for *any* injury, including those resulting from the known and normal risks of treatment.

Impaired physicians are by no means the only dangerous doctors—just the most numerous. And the medical community seems to be no more effective at rooting out the other categories than it is at dealing with its chemically impaired colleagues.

GROSS INCOMPETENTS

How even grossly incompetent physicians can skirt discipline by the medical establishment is shown by the case of Dr. Milos Klvana, reported by M. Carroll Thomas in *Medical Economics*. After receiving a medical degree in his native Czechoslovakia, Klvana did his internship in Virginia, then entered a residency program in New York City to train to become an obstetrician-gynecologist. He was dropped from this program after three years because of serious doubts about his competence. Among his problems, he had a tendency to use drugs to induce labor before first making sure the patient's pelvis could adequately support a normal delivery.

Klvana then entered an anesthesiology residency in California.

During the first year of his new training program, a young woman under Klvana's care died of cardiac arrest while having a tendon repaired. After one year in the program, Klvana was rated by his supervisors as "exceptional"—meaning exceptionally bad. Klvana resigned from the program and opened an office as a general practitioner in Valencia, California.

In 1978 Klvana had his first run-in with the law when he was caught by an undercover sting operation for providing drugs to detectives without first performing a medical examination. He pleaded guilty to twenty-six counts of improper prescribing and the Medical Board of California (then known as the Board of Medical Quality Assurance) placed him on probation for five years, limited his ability to prescribe addictive drugs, and placed him under supervision.

Questions about Klvana's competency continued. In 1980 a hospital where he practiced revoked his privileges and, to comply with California law, filed a report of its actions with the Board. A second hospital suspended his privileges and a third forced him to resign. These forced resignations were not reported to the Board. Klvana shifted much of his practice into his private offices, even advertising them as "birthing centers."

In 1982 Klvana sent an unlicensed midwife to the home of one of his patients in the early stages of labor. Despite the midwife's report that the delivery showed clear signs of complications, Klvana allowed the home delivery to continue. The baby quickly developed severe respiratory distress, and the midwife herself called another doctor for help. The second doctor told her to rush the baby to the hospital emergency department, but the baby died en route. The cause of death was RH-incompatibility, a condition that Klvana should have discovered earlier. The couple who lost this baby would have a second die also while under Klvana's care.

As the deaths and botched deliveries mounted up, so did the complaints about Klvana to the Board of Medicine. Yet none of these reports were brought before the Board when they met to consider the doctor's petition for an early end to his probation. The petition was granted in March 1983.

In October of 1983, another botched delivery in Klvana's office resulted in another dead infant. Klvana suggested to the parents that they bury the baby in their backyard and take a vacation to Hawaii with the money they would save by not requesting an autopsy. The parents complained to the Board and sued Klvana for malpractice. Although they eventually won a $1 million award against the doctor, they would collect nothing. Klvana had few assets and no malpractice insurance.

Finally, in February 1984, after the death of yet another baby at the hands of Klvana (there were at least nine infant deaths, although the exact number is not known because Klvana did not always file birth and death certificates), the hospital where the infant was pronounced dead contacted the Orange County District Attorney's Office.

The D.A.'s Office responded that they couldn't prosecute Klvana unless at least two medical experts were willing to testify that his care was criminally negligent. The Medical Board had one of its physicians investigate. Although the Board physician concluded that Klvana's treatment, "didn't differ from Third World quality care," that doctor declined to classify his care as "criminally negligent." The Board closed its case.

The D.A.'s Office, however, continued its investigation. Finally, in October 1986, they arrested Klvana for murder. By this time at least three more babies had died. Klvana remained in jail for more than a year before his bail was lowered to the point he could post it. While the Board of Medicine had begun proceedings to suspend Klvana's license, no formal action was ever taken. And while Klvana's own attorney had promised the court that his client would not practice medicine pending the outcome of the trial, Klvana ignored this request and resumed practice. This time, however, the D.A.'s office acted quickly and took Klvana back into custody.

At trial Klvana's own attorneys admitted their client was incompetent. Their chief defense was that a murder conviction requires intent to kill, and Klvana didn't know he was so incompetent that his treatment amounted to murder. Klvana was eventually found guilty on nine counts of second-degree murder, among other charges, and sentenced to fifty-three years in prison.

In response to public outcry, the California Board of Medicine performed an internal audit of its handling of the Klvana affair. It is a testament to the scope of the problem of self-policing in medicine that the Board found little fault with its own actions.

UNETHICAL PREDATORS

The Hippocratic oath is the oldest recorded statement of professional ethics. It recognizes that medicine, more than any other calling, requires that its practitioners be men and women of good moral character and behavior. Without this, the trust needed to create an effective doctor-patient relationship cannot be established.

Nonetheless, there are plenty of unethical physicians out there who use their power and authority to prey on their patients. For example, despite the fact that the Hippocratic oath and the AMA's Code of Ethics expressly forbid physicians from having sexual contact with their patients, this is a common source of patient complaints and malpractice suits, especially against psychiatrists. Because many patients are confused and shamed by the doctor's misconduct, they may endure years of abuse before they finally complain to the authorities. And even then, it's their word against the doctor's, and the law often sides with the doctor.

In 1960 a seventeen-year-old high school student identified in court records only as "N. N." saw Minnesota family physician Hideo D. Mori for problems that included irregular menstruation and cramps. Mori conducted a pelvic examination. Because the girl had never before received a gynecological exam, she did not know what it involved. During the examination Mori penetrated her vagina with his finger, explaining that she was "small" and needed to be stretched. During her next two visits, Mori also penetrated her with his finger.

Later that year, N. N. was hospitalized for bleeding ulcers. While she was in the hospital, Mori came to her private room and explained that her problems resulted from sexual frustration and an inability to reach orgasm. By way of "treatment," Mori massaged and kissed her breasts and again penetrated her with his finger.

Over the next two years, Mori repeatedly massaged the girl's clitoris and vagina, stating that this was necessary to prevent the return of her ulcers. At one point he attempted to penetrate her with his penis, stating that she needed to experience what a penis felt like. Mori continued to manipulate and abuse his patient in this way until 1982—a period of twenty-two years since the abuse had first begun.

N. N. was one of a number of women who filed sexual abuse complaints against Mori before the Minnesota State Medical Board revoked his license in 1987. And by the time N. N. worked through her emotional problems enough to confront Mori in court for malpractice, the statute of limitations had expired and her suit was dismissed.

PSYCHOPATHIC SERIAL KILLERS

Even when he was in medical school at Southern Illinois University, people thought Michael Swango was strange because of his obsessions with violent death and newspaper photos of car crashes. He also liked to talk about serial killers. But his classmates had no idea that he was about to become one.

Swango graduated from medical school in 1983 (after having been failed one year for making up patient histories) and then began his internship at the Ohio State University College of Medicine. Apparently his killing spree also began about this time. In 1985 he was convicted of poisoning six co-workers with insecticide and sentenced to five years in prison. He lost his medical license but, because none of the six died, he served only thirty months in prison. While he was serving his sentence, he was investigated for several mysterious patient deaths during his internship. Although several patients or their nurses had reported that patients had become acutely ill or died shortly after Swango administered "medication" to a patient, the officials in charge of the investigation concluded that there was not enough evidence to bring charges.

After his release from prison, Swango was accepted to a residency training program at the University of South Dakota in 1992. He was fired shortly thereafter when it was learned that he had lied about his criminal background on his application.

Using more lies and an alias, he was accepted into the psychiatry residency program at University Medical Center at Stony Brook, New York, in 1993. He disappeared from the program later that year after the FBI turned up to investigate the death of a patient who had lapsed into a coma shortly after Swango gave him a "sedative."

Swango then began practicing medicine in the African nation of Zimbabwe, then moved to neighboring Zambia. Facing murder charges following a string of at least six suspicious deaths in Zimbabwe, Swango fled in 1995. In 1997 he surfaced in Chicago, where he was arrested by the FBI.

In 1998 Swango pleaded guilty to perjury and was sent back to prison. In July 2000 just days before his scheduled release, federal prosecutors announced that Swango was being charged with killing three patients in a Long Island hospital in 1993. Swango pleaded guilty to the murder charges to avoid the death penalty. He was sentenced to three consecutive life sentences without the possibility of parole.

In his book *Blind Eye: How the Medical Establishment Let a Doctor Get Away with Murder* (Simon & Schuster), Pulitzer Prize–winning author

James Stewart presents a scathing attack on the medical establishment's failure to stop Swango in spite of eyewitness accounts of his murderous activities. He describes Swango as a psychopathic killer who is estimated to have murdered between thirty-five and sixty patients. According to Stewart, doctors were taken in by Swango's charm and good looks and refused to consider that he might be a murderer. They were further deterred by fears of liability, either by a lawsuit from Swango or by malpractice suits from his victims or their families. There was also concern about protecting the prestige of the institutions for which the doctors worked.

I think you'll agree with Ben Wilson, M.D., the Salem, Oregon, doctor involved in the fight against medical hucksters for many years who told me, "Good criminals are good at deception." And it's not just the doctors themselves who can be psychopathic killers. Sometimes it's their employees. The nationally publicized case of pediatric nurse Genene Jones in the early 1980s is an example.

Suspicion about Jones began to emerge in the early 1980s after eighty-two patients died over a two-and-a-half-year period in the pediatric intensive-care unit where she worked. Many of these deaths occurred under mysterious circumstances, often with no clear-cut cause. An epidemiologist (a scientist who studies the occurrence and spread of diseases) from the Centers for Disease Control in Atlanta was brought in to investigate. The timing of the deaths pointed squarely at Jones. The investigator found that a child in the unit was eleven times more likely to die when Jones was on duty than when she was not; further, a child was twenty-five times more likely to require cardiopulmonary resuscitation when Jones was present. And this pattern of unusual deaths on her shift continued even when Jones knew the investigation was focusing on her.

Despite this obvious statistical pattern, the university teaching hospital that housed the pediatric unit where Jones worked could find no conclusive evidence that she had caused the deaths. Not only were no criminal charges filed against Jones, the hospital took no action to stop her from practicing nursing. In 1982 she was allowed to resign from the hospital nursing staff with her license and her reputation intact.

That same year Jones took a position in the private offices of a local pediatrician. Within a one-month period six patients under Jones' care mysteriously quit breathing and underwent resuscitation. One baby died, and tests following the autopsy showed that she had been repeatedly injected with succinylcholine chloride, a fast-acting and powerful muscle relaxant resembling curare. It's usually indicated as an adjunct to general anesthesia and to facilitate tracheal insertion. The injections had paralyzed the girl's breathing muscles, leading to her death. The pediatrician had kept a supply of the drug in her office, and several doses were unaccountably missing. This was enough circumstantial evidence to lead to Jones' arrest. It also led to a reexamination of several of the other, previously unexplained deaths associated with her. In 1984 she was convicted of the girl's murder and sentenced to ninety-nine years in prison. She was later convicted of injecting a baby with heparin and sentenced to sixty years.

But what was the motive? Prosecutors speculate that Jones was seeking the "thrill" of taking charge of a life-threatening situation and the hero's status she received for bringing a child back from the brink of death. The fact that as many as forty-six children may have died when this ploy failed was, quite simply, a price she was willing to pay. Shortly after her conviction, it was rumored that several hospitals that had employed Jones over the years shredded her personnel files lest these records be used against them in malpractice actions covering mysterious deaths in their own pediatric wards.

PROTECTING YOURSELF

Your best defense against an impaired physician begins with a heightened awareness that a problem might exist. Watch out for it. Trust your basic instincts. You know what constitutes socially acceptable behavior. You know how doctors are supposed to act and talk. You know where, how, and under what circumstances they're supposed to touch you. In particular, remember that it is never, ever, *under any circumstances,* appropriate for your doctor to speak or behave toward you in a sexually suggestive manner.

Again, *trust your instincts:* If your doctor's behavior makes you uneasy, there's probably a good reason you're feeling the way you do. Your doctor is supposed to treat you with dignity and respect at all times. If he or she falls short in this department, find one who doesn't. Don't allow yourself to be cowed into assuming that, just because your doctor has been to medical school, whatever he or she says or does is acceptable.

You also know the signs of chemical impairment. Slurred speech, alcohol on the breath, difficulty in concentrating, and other symptoms of drug and alcohol abuse are well known. You may not normally think to watch for them in your physician, but you should.

Obviously, if you notice signs of impairment, it's time to find another doctor. But the process shouldn't end there. It's also important that you complain to the proper authorities. Everyone benefits—you, other patients, the medical community, and even the impaired physician—when such doctors are identified and placed into treatment programs.

The procedure for registering a complaint varies from one state to the next. In all cases the information will be kept strictly confidential and the doctor will never know the source or any other details of the complaint. Your best option is to call the state board of medical examiners in your state capital, or contact the Federation of State Medical Boards of the U.S. at 1-817-868-4000 for specific advice on registering your complaint. You may be referred to an 800 number or you may be asked to put your complaint in writing and mail it. In any case, keep your information as specific as possible. Instead of "Dr. Smith was drunk when he treated me last Saturday," tailor your comments: "When I was treated at Community Hospital on January third of this year, I smelled alcohol on Dr. Smith's breath and his speech seemed slurred." In that way, your information will be most useful to the authorities involved.

Likewise, a complaint along the lines of, "Dr. Smith sexually assaulted me during my pelvic examination," might leave the physicians who review it wondering if you really understood what a pelvic exam might entail. From such a vague statement it's not even clear whether you understood that a pelvic exam necessarily involves an inspection of the vagina. By contrast, stating that "Dr. Smith repeatedly stroked my clitoris while taking my Pap smear," makes it absolutely clear that the actions you are alleging were improper and unacceptable.

Another defense against impaired physicians is to routinely request second opinions before consenting to any major treatment, especially surgery requiring general anesthesia. No responsible physician would take offense at this, and many medical insurance companies already require it. Remember that a physician doesn't have to be intoxicated or "high" at the time of your treatment in order to suffer impaired judgment or performance. Seeking a second opinion will at least reduce the chance of your suffering through a needless surgery or other treatment. It also helps identify impaired physicians by bringing negligent medical care to the attention of other doctors. If a doctor sees repeated instances in which a colleague gives negligent diagnoses or proposes inappropriate treatments, that doctor is ethically—and sometimes legally—obliged to notify the hospital peer review committee or state board of medical examiners.

The problem of impaired physicians is much broader than is generally realized. It affects all of us, and we must all work together to solve it.

chapter 5

When "M.D." Means "Money Doctor"

Don' t Let Your Doctor Rip You Off

IN 1986 ELLEN BURSTEIN MACFARLANE was a respected investigative con-sumer reporter working for an Orlando, Florida, television station when her neurologist diagnosed the troubling weakness in her left leg as result-ing from MS. Multiple sclerosis is an incurable disease of the central nervous system that, in its most severe form, can leave its victims totally and permanently disabled. The doctor told MacFarlane that hers was a mild case, and encouraged her to go on with life as usual.

Although she carried on her reporting work, over the next five years her condition steadily deteriorated. By 1991 it had degenerated into the worst form of the disease, severe chronic progressive MS. By now she could only get around with the help of a walker or motorized scooter.

That May, MacFarlane received a burst of hope in the form of a magazine article sent to her by a friend. It was a copy of the March 18 issue of *New York* magazine, and the nine-page cover story was about a brilliant and charismatic physician by the name of Irving I. Dardik, M.D. Dardik had developed an elaborate theory centering on the idea that chronic diseases were the result of a decrease in heart-rate variability. Simply put, the more regular your heart rate, the more susceptible you would be to chronic disease.

To combat the problem, Dardik had developed a therapy he called "Superesonant Wavenergy." His claim was that, by quickly raising and lowering a patient's heart rate through exercise, he could correct imbalances in the immune system that cause MS, amyotrophic lateral sclerosis (ALS or Lou Gehrig's disease), chronic fatigue syndrome, and almost every other chronic disease.

As dubious as these theories might sound, Dardik's credentials alone were enough to give him credibility. He was a vascular surgeon (a doctor who operates on the blood vessels), an assistant professor at Albert Einstein College of Medicine, founding chairman of the U.S. Olympic Committee's Sports Medicine Council, and winner of the AMA's prestigious research award. People who would otherwise dismiss Dardik's theories as nonsensical were taken in by the doctor's stature in the medical community. MacFarlane was one of them. MacFarlane recounted her story in her book *Legwork: An inspiring journey through a chronic illness.*

MacFarlane arranged to meet with Dardik, and she immediately became a believer. Dardik enthusiastically told her that he had the answer to her problem. He insisted he would not simply put her into remission; he would cure her. And it would take only one year. But his treatments would not come easy or cheap. She would have to pay $100,000—half to be paid up front—and move to New York for several months.

Desperately believing in the promise that she could return to a normal life, MacFarlane convinced her family to help her raise the money. But seven months later, MacFarlane was worse off than ever. She was now confined to a wheelchair, needed twenty-four-hour nursing care and, worst of all, had to quit the job she loved. Needless to say, Dardik offered no restitution for his failed promises.

MacFarlane, however, was not done with Dardik. Unlike most victims of MediScammers, she was able to exact a certain level of revenge against the quack who stole her money plus something even more important—the precious last months of her physical independence. As a former consumer reporter, MacFarlane had made a living taking thieves and con artists to task. She knew what to do and how to do it. Thanks to her complaints to the medical licensing authorities, Dardik lost his medical licenses in New York and New Jersey, and was fined $40,000. She also sued Dardik for fraud, eventually settling out of court. Although she's not saying how much she recovered, she claims to be satisfied with the resolution.

Of course, MacFarlane can never recover the time and effort she spent in futile efforts to recuperate her failing body—time that a bright and ambitious woman like herself could have put to far better use had not the false hope of a cure been dangled in front of her.

THE BUSINESS OF MEDICINE

We should never lose sight of the fact that medicine, like almost every other venture in America, is a business—and well it should be. To become a doctor, one must first invest many years of hard work plus tens of thousands of dollars out-of-pocket. Physicians are entitled to make a good living from all that effort.

Another important point is that the profit motive makes American medicine the best in the world. In countries where the government provides medical care for free or at nominal cost, patients almost always must wait in line—sometimes for years—to receive non-emergency services; and even then health care is often rationed. For example, no one over age sixty-five is allowed a coronary bypass operation in the United Kingdom unless he or she has the resources to pay for it themselves.

As with any other business venture in America, doctors and hospitals compete against each other, and the prices are allowed to rise as high as the traffic will bear. But because even nonprofit institutions can set prices above their costs, providers of medically related services on every level have plenty of incentive to make those services readily available. Although we Americans may gripe about the high cost of our health care, we mustn't lose sight of what we get in return. Any of us who have medical insurance or other means to pay can get almost any service we want whenever we want it. And that's something few of us are willing to sacrifice in order to lower costs.

The problem, of course, is that the American way of practicing medicine also creates a lot of greed. Even competent and otherwise conscientious doctors are by no means immune to the siren song of the almighty dollar. And sometimes it's the other physicians who get fed up with it. Take the case of the Ohio internal medicine specialist who made so much money from Medicare patients that fellow doctors on his hospital staff turned him in to the authorities. Since defrauding Medicare is a federal crime, Medicare sent its investigators to inspect the doctor's records. They compared his hospital chart notes with chart notes of patients he had seen in his office, along with those he saw in a nursing home he serviced. The investigators found that the internist often claimed to be at two or three different locations at the same time. The day after he was confronted with this evidence, the doctor disappeared— presumably having fled the country to avoid prosecution.

There are many ways that a doctor or hospital can rip off you or your insurance company. One way, as with Dr. Dardik, is to invent a bogus cure that only the inventor offers. With no competition, the inventor can set his own price for the treatments. And if you complain that you're not getting better . . . Well, says the doctor, the cure works 90 percent of the time and you just happen to be that unlucky one patient in ten on whom it doesn't work; and, of course, there's no way of knowing how many other patients the doctor may have told the same thing.

Even medically accepted treatments can be, and frequently are, used under fraudulent circumstances. For example, until recently, doctors could legally refer patients to laboratories, physical therapy centers, and other facilities in which the doctor held a financial interest. In 1992 the *New England Journal of Medicine* published a study reporting, among other things, that doctors who held a financial stake in laboratories or other facilities used those facilities 60 percent more often than physicians who did not hold such investments. Although the federal government tightened regulations in order to clamp down on such conflicts of interest, greedy physicians simply found other ways to make a quick buck at the expense of their patients. Following are just a few examples.

DRUG STUDIES

In the summer of 1995 an elderly woman from Whittier, California, was suffering from high blood pressure. Her physician, family practitioner Robert Fiddes, enrolled her in a clinical trial of a new anti-hypertensive (blood pressure–lowering) drug named Cozaar. But instead of dropping the woman's blood pressure, the Cozaar caused it to rise to dangerous levels. The registered nurse, who was the coordinator of the study and an employee of Fiddes, sent the patient back to the doctor, urging that she be dropped from the study immediately.

Fiddes, however, had other ideas. He placed his patient on two other drugs meant to lower her blood pressure and kept her on the study. Not only was this a violation of the drug company's rule that patients in the study could not be taking other medications, but it made it impossible to sort out the effects of Cozaar from those of the other two drugs.

Good research wasn't the only victim of this fraud. A few days later, the patient returned to the doctor's office with a bruised face, slurred speech, and difficulty in walking. She told the study coordinator that she had passed out while bathing. The nurse took the woman's pulse and found that her heart was barely beating—the presumed result of being overmedicated with anti-hypertensive drugs.

When the nurse again requested that the woman be dropped from the study, Fiddes refused again. The woman was kept on the medications for several more weeks. Eventually she wound up in a hospital under the care of another doctor for treatment of her problems, and the nurse resigned from her job in disgust. As for Fiddes, he pocketed a hefty payment from the drug company as a reward for keeping the patient in his study.

Fiddes, who became the centerpiece of an extensive *New York Times* exposé by Kurt Eichenwald and Gina Kolata, participated in almost two hundred drug company–sponsored research studies. With physician reimbursement typically running between $40,000 and $50,000 per study, he probably took in between $8 to $10 million for his participation—and that was on top of the regular income from his practice. Not only were inappropriate patients placed in these studies, but patient data—and sometimes even the patients themselves—were fabricated. Fiddes' staff ran electrocardiograms and other tests on each other, substituting these results for those of the patient when the patient failed to meet the guidelines for inclusion in the study. Bottles of urine and blood plasma that fit the criteria the drug companies were looking for were also kept in a refrigerator in Fiddes' offices. When the patient's own fluids failed to match the required criteria, Fiddes simply had his staff substitute the stored samples for those of the patient. Patients weren't even asked if they wanted to take part in the studies—they were simply enrolled as guinea pigs and told what to do.

Eventually the law caught up with Fiddes when a disgruntled former employee complained of Fiddes' monumental fraud directly to the FDA. When his remaining employees agreed to cooperate with federal investigators, Fiddes himself felt compelled to plea-bargain. In return for a reduced prison sentence of fifteen months for fraud and conspiracy, Fiddes showed the investigators just how easy it was to manufacture and submit fraudulent research data.

Fiddes maintained that fraud was rampant in the drug-research industry. He may be right. Certainly, as a follow-up article in the *New York Times* showed, the huge financial incentives that drug companies pay doctors for recruiting and monitoring human guinea pigs can create a conflict of interest between the patients' welfare and the physician's paycheck. And, as the Fiddes case shows, it isn't always the patient who wins.

Another concern: If research fraud really is becoming more common, then the safety and efficacy of the newer drugs coming into the market also may be called into question.

It wasn't always this way. Until the early 1990s, most studies for testing new drugs were conducted at medical schools and university centers. The drug companies paid the universities directly for these services, and the tests were conducted by salaried faculty members who received no direct payments or other kickbacks for their participation. Fraudulent and sloppy research still happened, of course, but there were few financial incentives to encourage such practices.

The economics of drug testing began to change when HMOs and other managed-care plans began squeezing drug makers to lower their prices on existing medications. The manufacturers, aided by FDA changes that allowed for quicker approval of new drugs, responded by rushing the development of newer pharmaceuticals that carried higher profit margins.

The medical schools, however, were unable to cope with the flood of new drug studies now demanded by the manufacturers. So the drug companies turned to a new source—doctors in private practice. Today, virtually any licensed physician can participate in clinical trials of new drugs, which means that any patient, knowingly or not, can become a guinea pig.

Aside from the fact that it is highly unethical to involve patients in such studies without their knowledge or permission, there is the issue of safety. In most cases, there are drugs already in existence that can effectively treat the patient's problem. Yet in clinical investigations, such patients are given drugs that may or may not be effective at all. Even worse, about half of the patients are given placebos, or sham medications that contain no active ingredients. The bottom line is that, even when the study is conducted flawlessly, the patients are put at risk. Too often the only beneficiary of such studies is the doctor's pocketbook.

Nor are the drug companies themselves above misconduct in the use of medical research. In 1996 the *Wall Street Journal* ran a report about the synthetic thyroid hormone Synthroid. When Synthroid came on the market in 1958, the FDA approved it without first demanding research data to support its effectiveness. Synthroid quickly became the drug of choice for treating hypothyroidism (a condition in which the patient's own thyroid doesn't produce enough hormone), and in 1996 accounted for 84 percent of the $600 million Americans spent every year on thyroid-replacement products. Although there are much cheaper generic thyroid-replacement products now on the market, they've traditionally been stuck in a Catch-22 situation. In order to get doctors to prescribe the generics, they must first prove that the generics are as effective as Synthroid. But since Synthroid was introduced without prior clinical trials, there was no data for the generics to compare themselves with.

Still, the rivals persisted and gradually began to erode the virtual monopoly held by Synthroid. Boots, the British company that was manufacturing Synthroid at the time, paid $250,000 to researchers with the University of California to compare Synthroid with its three biggest rivals. To the chagrin of Boots, the researchers found that the generics were every bit as effective as Synthroid and would save American thyroid patients $356 million a year. Even worse for Boots, the research had been written up and accepted for publication by *JAMA*—and right at the time Boots was preparing to sell itself to BASF. But Boots had an easy out. Their contract with the UC researchers forbade publication of the study data without Boots' permission. Naturally the company denied permission for publication, and Synthroid continued to flourish as the third-most-prescribed drug in the United States.

In 1997, over the protest of the manufacturer, *JAMA* published the results of the study. BASF's subsidiary, Knoll Pharmaceuticals, claimed the study was flawed and the results invalid. In May 1997 a class action suit was filed against the manufacturer for overcharging consumers during the seven years the research hadn't been released.

Fast-forward to 1999. The attorneys general of thirty-seven states alleged that Knoll Pharmaceuticals had broken the law by claiming Synthroid was better than its competition. These allegations were based in part on charges that Knoll tried to interfere in the publication of the results of its study. Knoll agreed to pay the thirty-seven states a total of $48 million. They agreed to stop making deceptive claims in the future. Earlier that same year, a report from the U.S. House Government Reform and Oversight Committee revealed that seniors paid $27.05 per month for Synthroid, which was over 1,400 percent *more* than the $1.75 paid by favored group purchasers such as HMOs and hospitals, according to author Mary Shoman.

On August 8, 2000, the Synthroid class action lawsuit settlement was approved. Knoll estimated that almost 780,000 consumers would receive payments of approximately $74 to $111 each if no appeals were filed.

UNNECESSARY SERVICES

When a doctor tells us we need a particular service or procedure, we naturally assume that the recommendation or treatment is made in our best interests. Unfortunately, sometimes such decisions are made on the basis of what is best for the physician's bottom line. In May 1998 orthopedic surgeon (bone doctor) Harold F. Goodman of Massachusetts was indicted for subjecting nineteen patients on Medicaid to over two thousand unnecessary medical tests and procedures, resulting in a profit to him of over $100,000 in fraudulent Medicaid reimbursements.

According to the indictments, Goodman repeatedly administered injections of steroids into the joints of his patients, for which Medicaid paid him $60 each, and then took X rays for which he was paid another $20 to $40 each. Steroids are powerful drugs that can have many undesirable side effects, including softening of the bones, called osteoporosis. On average the patients received an injection every week and an X ray every two weeks. Some patients received more than eighty injections and over fifty X rays during a three-year period from July 1992 through June 1995. According to an outside panel of orthopedic surgeons who reviewed the charts of these patients, neither the X rays nor the injections served any real medical purpose and exposed the patients needlessly to excessive radiation plus the considerable risk of side effects from the steroid injections. Goodman was charged with seventy-six counts of Medicaid fraud. In April 2000 Goodman received a six-month jail sentence and $62,500 fine after being convicted on thirteen counts.

Physicians aren't the only ones who get accused of delivering unnecessary services. For the TV show *Extra,* I took along a hidden camera to see just how far some chiropractors would go in treating a painless, nonexistent injury. First I had a thorough exam by licensed chiropractor Jennifer Sellars, D.C. (doctor of chiropractic). She took X rays, which I would show to other chiropractors. Her examination showed me to be in perfect health.

Then I made appointments to be examined by several chiropractors. My story was that I'd fallen off a treadmill. I felt fine—no pain, no swelling or stiffness. I just wanted to be checked out before I resumed exercising.

I was examined by chiropractor Margaret Colucci, D.C. "Don't fix what's not broken," she told me. She, like half the chiropractors I visited, told me I was fine and didn't need care. The other half had differing opinions.

After viewing my X rays, a third chiropractor tested my muscle reactions. She said I'd pulled some muscles. As I was lying down, she asked me to look at my right foot, which she claimed was pointing north. "That's dramatic," she said. Her diagnosis was "a sprain/strain of the low back and right foot." For this, she estimated that I would need two months of treatment at an approximate cost of $1,016.

The fourth chiropractor gave me a physical exam lasting only a minute or so, then diagnosed a "loss of lumbar normal range of motion especially in the lateral bending" on the right side. Fixing it would require twice-weekly treatments for four to six weeks. The cost of twelve treatments would be approximately $1,200.

The fifth chiropractor gave me an extensive examination. He asked me if I was having a lot of pain. I told him no. He said my spine was generally in good health, but that "you've got a little imbalance in your pelvis." His diagnosis: "traumatic lumbosacral joint dysfunction and traumatic intervertebral disc injury." He prescribed three visits a week for three to four months. Estimated cost of treatment—about $5,000.

I showed my undercover videos to Jennifer Sellars. Her reaction: "I was angry. I was shocked. And there were points I started laughing, it was so preposterous." She reiterated that any chiropractor who had prescribed treatment was out of line. Said Sellars, "You repeated yourself—you had no signs or symptoms, no pain, no swelling, no inflammation, no loss of anything. They still came up with that sprain/strain diagnosis, which can only happen from an injury." An injury I didn't have.

I went back to the third chiropractor and told her who I was and that I hadn't fallen off a treadmill and didn't have any injuries. She said that didn't surprise her, but that she could find injuries to muscles that had occurred as long as sixty years ago. And according to the way she tests, I had a muscle injury. She then informed me it was her lunch hour and she wanted to take it. End of interview.

I then confronted the fourth chiroprator with the same revelation. His response: "I think you would benefit from treatment. I'm okay with that."

The fifth chiropractor, who wanted $5,000 to treat my nonexistent injury, became quite hostile when confronted with my true story. When he denied finding trauma after examining me, I showed him a copy of his written diagnosis. That only enraged him further. He said, "I understand what that says. That's based on history. Where it came from, I told you in there, I don't know. And you can't argue with that."

I replied, "The experts have said that I don't have a spinal injury."

To this he countered, "You know what? I'm done with you. You can leave now. You can leave now. Turn that camera off."

Following my investigation, the fifth chiropractor left his practice.

Dentists, too, have been known to offer unneeded services. Jon Kent Dezelle, a Beaumont, Texas, dentist in the mid-1990s, collected more than $500,000 a year from the state's Medicaid program, in addition to his regular practice income. In 1994 alone, Dezelle installed 2,526 stainless-steel crowns—and did not do a single filling—on the baby teeth of children on Medicaid. A crown pays three times more than a single filling. Not all of Dezelle's colleagues agreed that his methods were appropriate.

In one case Dezelle recommended that a child on Medicaid receive eight crowns and two pulpotomies. A pulpotomy is a root canal on a baby tooth. He also insisted that the child would have to undergo general anesthesia at an outpatient surgical center—which would pay the dentist $75 more than using an in-office local anesthetic. The mother, concerned that Dezelle's recommendations seemed a little extreme, sought a second opinion. She found a dentist who gave the child two crowns, filled three teeth, and did two pulpotomies, all using a local anesthetic. The total savings to the taxpayers was about $1,000.

When a fraud investigator working for the state's Medicaid carrier began questioning the practices of Dezelle and other dentists who were making big bucks on Medicaid, the dentists complained and got the investigator—who was himself a dentist—fired. But by then Dezelle had attracted the attention of prosecutors. In 1999 Dezelle settled a fraud action against him by agreeing to repay the state and federal governments over $500,000 for providing medically unnecessary dental services to children. Dezelle admitted no wrongdoing in agreeing to the settlement.

Sometimes it's not even the doctor or dentist who is responsible for the delivery of unnecessary services. A Michigan laboratory came under scrutiny of Medicare investigators when an employee reported that the laboratory routinely charged Medicare and Medicaid for diagnostic tests that had not been ordered by a physician—a violation of federal regulations. The resulting fraud investigation identified over $1.6 million in false claims that the laboratory had submitted for Medicare and Medicaid patients. In 1998 the laboratory agreed to a settlement in which it would shell out $6.8 million in repayments and fines.

UNDELIVERED SERVICES

In 1994 Los Angeles general practitioner Davoud Yedidsion billed more house calls to Medicare than any other physician in California. In an era when few doctors make house calls anymore, that seemed to be an admirable record. But a closer look at his patient base immediately began to reveal problems. For example, some of the patients he claimed to be treating had been dead for years. Others were confined to nursing homes, and some had even been incarcerated in state mental institutions.

The U.S. Department of Health and Human Services sent in fraud investigators, who turned up even more irregularities. The doctor had submitted bills for patients who were confined to nursing homes that had barred Yedidsion from their premises. Other patients steadfastly denied that Yedidsion had ever treated them. In all, according to the investigators, the doctor had submitted over 1,600 false bills to Medicare from 1992 through 1995, for which he was paid over $300,000. In November 1998 Yedidsion pled guilty to Medicare fraud. He received a two-year sentence and was fined $361,000.

Medicaid and Medicare fraud are big business. In 1996, according to the government's own figures, Medicare spent over $23.2 billion—about 14 percent of its total budget—on payments for "inappropriate" patient services. About $5 billion of those funds were paid to physicians. Although these numbers have recently declined thanks to government crackdowns on fraud, abuse, and waste, in 1998 the government still estimated that 7.1 percent of all Medicare payments, amounting to $12.6 billion, were spent inappropriately. And just how outrageous this kind of fraud can be is illustrated by the case of a medical management company in Texas. In what the Texas Comptroller of Public Accounts ridiculed as "extraordinary measures to keep someone alive," the company continued to bill the state's Medicaid program for services supposedly provided by an elderly staff physician for years after the doctor had become incapacitated, and continued billing for his services for several months after the doctor had died.

Even pharmacists have been known to bill for undelivered services. In 1998, Wisconsin pharmacist Jeffrey A. Wejrowski and his corporation were convicted of fraud after billing Medicaid for thirteen doses of a drug called Neupogen supposedly delivered to a nun at a nearby convent. Wejrowski did not actually furnish the drug, and knew that the nun was no longer using it after the convent had returned an unused dose. Neupogen is used to treat the side effects of chemotherapy, and Medicaid reimbursed the pharmacist almost $3,000 for each dose—that totaled up to more than $38,000 for medication that was never delivered. Wejrowski was ordered to repay more than $43,000 in restitution and serve eight months in jail.

UNSCRUPULOUS BILLING PRACTICES

More common than billing for undelivered services is the practice called "upcoding." That's when the doctor actually treats the patient, but bills the government or insurance company for a more intensive—and thus better-paying—level of service than was actually provided. For example, one psychiatrist billed every patient visit as one hour of individual psychotherapy. This applied to all patients, including those in group therapy as well as those he saw only for a few minutes while making rounds at the hospital. When a review of the doctor's billing practices revealed that he was billing for more than twenty-four hours per day of services, the fraud investigators were sent in. The courts slapped the psychiatrist with nearly $70 million in fines and repayments.

Another fraudulent practice is called "unbundling." That's when the doctor, instead of billing for a complete set of services, breaks them down into several separate actions for the purpose of increasing the payment. Assume, for example, a patient comes in with a broken arm. Normally the entire process of X-raying the arm, reading the X ray, setting the arm, and applying a cast to it would be bundled together and billed as a single service. Billing separately for each of those steps would be considered "unbundling."

Although this particular form of fraud doesn't normally affect the patient's actual care, sometimes it does. A Denver-based consultant who specializes in training physicians to bill appropriately for their services noted that a prospective client, a surgeon, did a lot of breast biopsies. The consultant asked the surgeon why he would have a patient come in one day to have her left breast biopsied, then have her return several days later to have her right breast done. The surgeon replied that Medicare paid him more money to do the breast biopsies separately than to do them both on the same day. The consultant informed the surgeon that he was committing fraud and refused to take him on as a client. A few months later, the surgeon was indicted for Medicare fraud.

KICKBACKS

In 1980 a Colorado Springs cardiologist was outraged when a salesman of cardiac pacemakers offered the doctor $500 for each time he would remove a competitor's pacemaker from a patient and replace it with one the salesman was promoting. The salesman's offer was not only unethical, but illegal, since it constituted a bribe. The irate doctor evicted the salesman, then notified Medicare, which pays for the installation of the majority of pacemakers in the U.S. Ultimately this led to a congressional investigation which uncovered "The Great Pacemaker Scandal."

It seems that not all of the doctor's colleagues had found the offer as offensive as he did. The pacemaker company had over four hundred salespeople, some making over $1 million per year, who were giving physicians bribes, kickbacks, and free vacations in return for preferential treatment of the company's products.

Certainly the company had its own financial incentives. It was charging Medicare $3,425 each for the pacemakers, three times more than it was charging Europeans for the same device. The pacemakers themselves involved technology that was no more complicated than that of an electronic watch; nor were they much more expensive to manufacture.

Even more disturbing was the fact that, in response to the financial incentives, doctors with very little knowledge or training in the use of pacemakers were installing the devices without ever having witnessed the installation procedure firsthand themselves. At times, the salesperson actually directed the operation. And a lot of pacemaker recipients—estimates range from 30 to 75 percent of them—didn't need the device in the first place. According to one estimate, over 200,000 Americans had pacemakers needlessly installed by 1983. This tremendous waste of money doesn't even take into account the loss in the quality of life of those healthy individuals who were forced to bear the physical and financial burdens of unnecessary surgery. Finally, how could a patient not live in constant fear of the pacemaker malfunctioning?

COMBATING MEDICAL GREED

The fight against medical greed begins with the simple awareness that not everyone who provides medical services to you—be it a doctor, nurse, pharmacist, chiropractor, or laboratory—always has your best interests at heart. Shop for health care the same way you would for a used car. Pay attention, be cautious of believing any promises, and don't hesitate to look elsewhere if you're not comfortable with the people you're dealing with.

Be especially wary of anyone offering "experimental" or "alternative" therapies or cures. Do some research before you start paying for what may be a bogus cure that is not only expensive but may prevent or delay you from seeking more effective care. Legitimate medical cures or treatments don't just pop out of thin air. Even the most brilliant clinical researcher builds on the ideas of colleagues, and those colleagues will test and refine those ideas even further. The result is a trail of published research in scientific and medical journals. And you can follow that trail and evaluate the research yourself. If you don't have a medical library nearby, you can access the National Library of Medicine's PubMed service online at www.ncbi.nlm.nih.gov/PubMed/. The site provides a search engine that allows you to look up recent articles on almost any medically related topic using keywords. Although you usually can't download entire articles, most come with an abstract or a summary that you can access online.

If you can't find a reference to the treatment in question—"experimental" or not—in the National Library of Medicine database, there's a very good chance that it's bogus. Don't for one minute believe the quack who complains that his or her research is being "suppressed" by the medical community. That doesn't happen. The science of medicine is, by its very nature, always open to new ideas. The fact that someone's theories about a cure or treatment aren't being published in the medical literature simply means that the ideas aren't being presented or investigated in a way that will withstand scientific scrutiny. If all you can find on a treatment is anecdotal evidence and testimonials, beware. That should be your first clue that it may be a sham.

If a cure or treatment presents a legitimate medical breakthrough, the financial rewards almost always will be enough to warrant having other physicians test the product and prove its efficacy in clinical trials. After all, if such a treatment is accepted by the mainstream medical community, the inventor stands to make much, much more money than if he or she is the only one offering it. So be extremely wary of anyone who offers an "exclusive" treatment that you can't get anywhere else.

Likewise, if your doctor invites you to take part in a study of a new drug, keep your eyes open and ask questions. And run for the door if the physician begins pressuring you or bristles at your questions.

An important question to consider when deciding whether to participate in clinical trials is whether or not there are already drugs on the market that can treat your condition safely and effectively. Often drug companies introduce new drugs not because they offer clear-cut advantages over existing treatments but because the patent has expired on the older drugs so that they are now available in the cheaper generic form. Newer drugs can be patented, meaning that the company who develops the drug can market it exclusively—which also means selling it at a premium price. That's good for the drug company's bottom line, but it doesn't mean that the drug being tested is even potentially better for you than one that's already on pharmacy shelves.

Always keep in mind that "newer" is not always better for you, the patient. After all, that's why the FDA insists in the first place that new drugs be tested clinically before they are released. If an older, effective treatment exists for your condition, do you want to risk taking a newer, less-understood drug—or maybe even a placebo—to achieve the same result? Do the potential benefits of the newer drug really outweigh the known or potential risks? Remember that doctors are paid to recruit patients into new drug studies, regardless of whether the medication under study is the best choice for the patient. So ask questions and make sure you fully understand the risks involved before you agree to be a human guinea pig.

Finally, examine the "explanation of benefits" statement you get from Medicare, Medicaid, or your private insurance company after treatment or hospitalization. Are all of the charges justified? Did all of the treatments or physician visits listed on the statement actually take place? If the charges aren't justified, there's usually a phone number given on the statement for you to call and complain. Do it. That's the only way we as patients can do our part to control medical greed and price-gouging.

chapter 6

Lying with Science

Just Because They Tell You It's "Scientifically Proven" Doesn't Mean It Is

YOU'RE AT A BAR and have had a couple too many to drink. Worried about getting a DWI while driving home? No problem—just go to the vending machine in the restroom, and for a buck-fifty you buy a packet of Neutralizer herbal capsules. According to the capsule manufacturer's promotional literature:

A study done by Harvard Medical School found that the herb Pueraria guards against the toxic side effects of alcohol consumption. Pueraria is the primary ingredient in the herbal formula called Alcohol Neutralizer. This product combines Pueraria and fourteen other herbs that help to rapidly detoxify the system of alcohol thus lowering ones' alcohol level.

Those claims were actually made by a Florida-based company that recruited entrepreneurs at $4,500 a pop to distribute their vending machines and Neutralizer capsules for sale in public restrooms. The sheer recklessness and outrageousness of these claims becomes obvious when one goes back and reads the original research upon which they are based. Researchers at Harvard Medical School did indeed investigate the effects of pueraria on alcohol metabolism in the early 1990s. The findings of this research, however, were almost diametrically opposed to the

Neutralizer claims. Far from detoxifying alcohol and speeding its removal from the body, the researchers found that pueraria actually *blocks* the breakdown of alcohol and produces a buildup of toxic aldehydes in the bloodstream. In this way, it acts similar to the anti-alcoholism drug Antabuse, which reacts with alcohol to make the patient violently ill, thus encouraging abstinence from alcohol consumption. In fact, pueraria is used by traditional Chinese herbalists for exactly this purpose. Instead of sobering up those who have had too much to drink, the herb has the potential of sending them to a hospital emergency room.

Nonetheless, my television camera team and I decided to put Neutralizer to the test. Under the supervision of Tim Dickerson, a police officer, six members of our team each had four shots of alcohol over a twenty-minute period. Their blood alcohol was measured by a Breathalyzer immediately after consuming the alcohol. Half of them then took Neutralizer capsules and the other half did not. After an hour, everyone took a Breathalyzer test again. It was found that everyone's blood alcohol had decreased by about the same amount, whether they had taken the Neutralizer or not. And most of the test subjects were still legally intoxicated. Although no one got ill from the herbs, we did notice a pronounced flushing on the faces of two of those who had taken the Neutralizer. According to the *Physician's Desk Reference,* facial flushing is an early sign of aldehyde toxicity.

The worst part of this MediScam is that it encourages people who might otherwise realize that they are too drunk to drive to falsely believe the herbs have "detoxified" them enough to get behind the wheel of a car. And what did the promoters of Neutralizer have to say about this? When confronted on camera, they flatly admitted they had never fully tested their herbal concoction to determine whether it lived up to their claims. But what about the potential tragedy that might result from a drunk driver? According to one of the promoters, "What if it works? What if it doesn't? Who knows? I don't owe anything to anybody."

Even though the promoter didn't believe she owed anything to anyone, the FTC disagreed. It charged the operators of the Florida-based companies marketing the Alcohol Neutralizer franchises with making deceptive and misleading claims about the product, and with violating the FTC's Franchise Rule by failing to provide basic disclosure and earnings claims documents. Although the defendants did not admit any wrongdoing, they paid an estimated $64,000 to settle the charges against them.

A LITTLE BIT OF SCIENCE—A Lot of Hocus-Pocus

One of the most frequent ploys of MediScammers is to start with a kernel of legitimate scientific knowledge or theory, then extrapolate it far past what the evidence—or even common sense—can reasonably justify. Another popular ploy is to legitimize a MediScam with "scientific studies" that have been either totally fabricated or published in dubious "medical journals" that are themselves owned by and run for the benefit of MediScammers. This false appearance of scientific authenticity is sometimes enough to convince even well-intentioned physicians that the claims are legitimate.

It's important to realize here that many MediScams are run by people with authentic medical degrees. And some of them honestly believe that they are offering legitimate tests or treatments. It's also important to realize that, while practicing medicine without a license is a crime, in many states simply using the letters "M.D." after your name is not. Thus, the person with a fictitious medical degree who gives public nutrition lectures under the name of "John Jones, M.D." in order to tout the need for his high-priced vitamin concoctions may not be committing a crime as long as he isn't actually diagnosing or treating diseases.

But no matter how persuasive the MediScammer's claims may be, the end result is that they will separate you from your money. What follows is only a partial catalog of some recent schemes that have used bad or even bogus science to make their products and services appear legitimate.

AN "ALTERNATIVE" CANCER TREATMENT

In 1991 Christina Stephanie Doek (not her real name) was diagnosed with uterine cancer and underwent a hysterectomy at a New York City hospital. Examination of the cancer showed that the cells were poorly differentiated. Generally, the more poorly differentiated the cancer cells, the more easily they can spread, or metastasize, to other parts of the body. Although there were no clear signs that Doek's cancer had, in fact, metastasized, her physicians recommended a course of radiation and chemotherapy to kill any cancer cells remaining in her system.

Having witnessed the suffering of a relative who had undergone chemotherapy, Doek decided to seek a second opinion. She met with Nicholas J. Gonzalez, a Flushing, New York, family practitioner. Although he had graduated from a traditional medical school, Gonzalez specialized in alternative therapies. Doek had learned about him by attending one of his lectures and listening to his tapes.

Gonzalez convinced Doek not to "mess" with radiation and chemotherapy. Instead, he put her on his own protocol, which included a special diet and six coffee enemas a day. Gonzalez assured his patient that he had a 75 percent success rate treating patients with her condition. According to Doek, Gonzalez never told her that he was not an oncologist (a cancer specialist) or that his protocol was experimental and not accepted by the mainstream medical community. He also told her that a special hair test he had devised showed there were still cancer cells in her body. This was something that even the physicians at the hospital had been unable to detect for sure.

Doek followed the protocol religiously for the next seven months. She was encouraged when Gonzalez assured her that his hair tests showed a steady reduction of the number of cancer cells in her body.

By June of 1992, however, Doek began experiencing back pain and failing vision. She discontinued the protocol and returned to the hospital. There it was discovered that the cancer had metastasized to her spine, a condition which eventually left her blind and bedridden.

Doek sued Gonzalez for malpractice—alleging that he had negligently persuaded her to forgo conventional therapy that would most likely have cured her cancer—and for lack of informed consent. The informed-consent claim alleged that she would not have consented to the protocol had she known it was of no therapeutic benefit. At the trial Dock presented expert testimony stating that the hair test for cancer cells was completely bogus and that the dietary regimen, if anything, encouraged the growth of cancer cells. The doctors who testified on her behalf painted Gonzalez as an out-and-out charlatan. Gonzalez countered that patients had a right to choose unconventional therapies, and that finding against him would put alternative practitioners out of business. He did not present a single witness to support the validity of his treatment.

The jury found the patient 49 percent at fault and the physician 51 percent at fault and awarded Doek over $4 million in compensatory damages and $150,000 in punitive damages. Gonzalez appealed, and the appellate court wrestled with the concept of what constitutes "informed consent." In reviewing previous legal decisions, the court determined that, in giving informed consent, the patient must first be given "appropriate" information. After all, a patient cannot be expected to know more or even as much about a treatment as a physician. Therefore, the patient must rely on information provided by the doctor in making a decision. And if the patient consents to treatment based on false or misleading information supplied by the physician, then the patient has not really consented to treatment at all. The appellate court upheld the verdict in its entirety.

HAIR ANALYSIS

It has long been known that minerals from the body are deposited in growing hair. As such, hair can be used as a screening device for minerals that should not be there at all, especially the heavy and highly poisonous metals mercury, lead, cadmium, and arsenic. But there is no clear and consistent relationship between the concentration of a mineral found in the hair and the blood level of that same mineral; therefore it is useless to try to diagnose high or low levels of essential nutrients like iron, calcium, magnesium, and so on from hair content. And it is totally fraudulent to claim that vitamin deficiencies can be diagnosed by this technique, since the hair is reduced to ash during mineral analysis, totally destroying any vitamins that might be present.

Yet the claims made by so-called practitioners who offer hair analysis can be absolutely astounding. In 1980 the Los Angeles City Attorney's Office prosecuted Benjamin and Sarah Colimore, owners of a health food store, after they claimed to have diagnosed a bad heart valve, abscesses of the pancreas, and benign growths of the liver, intestine, and stomach in a customer—all based on analysis of her hair. The Colimers prescribed two substances for their customer, one of which was an "herbal tea" that turned out to be nothing more than milk sugar, the other a milk-sugar product that contained traces of arsenic. The Colimores eventually pleaded no contest to charges of practicing medicine without a license, but were given only a $2,000 fine, suspended jail sentences, and two years of probation.

There are numerous sites on the Internet offering hair analysis. One I especially love reassuringly states that analysis of the hair does not have to be painful. Most include a questionnaire related to your health, diet, and lifestyle. For $40 to $50 and a lock of hair, you'll receive information about—guess what?—your health, diet, and lifestyle!

One thing is virtually certain: If you submit to a hair analysis by a chiropractor or "nutritional consultant," you will be diagnosed with at least a couple—more likely a myriad—of nutritional deficiencies or other health problems that he or she claims can be cured or treated by nutritional supplementation. And the person who "diagnosed" these deficiencies will charge you a small fortune for correcting them. If anyone ever offers you a hair analysis for anything beyond a screening for heavy-metal poisoning, you're about to be MediScammed.

WEIGHT LOSS SCHEMES—The Ideal MediScam

In theory, obesity should be one of the simplest diseases to treat. You simply convince the patient to take in less calories than he or she burns up every day, then let the laws of thermodynamics take over. In practice, however, obesity is one of the most difficult conditions to treat, and only a small number of patients who succeed in losing weight manage to keep it off for more than a few months.

The frustration of patients who are trying to lose weight makes them an ideal target for MediScammers because, at present, there are no cures for obesity that are both easy and legitimate. This creates a void in the marketplace, and there are plenty of hucksters claiming to have found the "magic" cure that will fill it. And they make a living off people who are so desperate for a way to melt pounds off effortlessly that they'll jump at almost anything, no matter how far-fetched. Case in point: In the early 1980s a mail-order outfit advertised special eyeglasses for dieters to wear while eating. The claim was that, because the lenses of the glasses were different colors, the brain became "disoriented" while eating and turned off the body's hunger signals quicker. The eyeglasses, which sold for around $15, had cardboard frames with one blue lens and one red lens. That's right—they were the same glasses theaters gave to patrons for viewing 3-D movies.

Although there was no scientific basis whatever for the eyeglass scam, a lot of the more convincing MediScams actually do have a scientific basis—or so it seems. A closer analysis reveals that even major drug companies may not be above disregarding science when it benefits their bottom line.

Good Science, Bad Communications—The Fen-Phen Story

In the early 1980s medical investigators working on the antidepressant drug Prozac discovered a link between serotonin and eating disorders. Serotonin is a naturally occurring neurotransmitter (a substance that helps nerves communicate with each other) found in the blood, and an increase in serotonin levels promotes a sense of well-being which helps shut off the appetite. Because Prozac inhibited the body's ability to remove serotonin from the blood, an unintended side effect of the drug was that many patients taking it lost weight. This led to the development of appetite-suppressing drugs specifically designed to block the body's serotonin-uptake mechanism. The most effective of these was dexfenfluramine (the "fen" in fen-phen), marketed under the brand name Redux. A close chemical cousin of Redux is fenfluramine, marketed under the brand name Pondimin.

From the outset it was realized that Redux should not be prescribed in combination with other drugs that affect serotonin metabolism. The body has two mechanisms for controlling serotonin levels: absorption into the platelets of the blood, which use it for clotting, and the serotonin-destroying enzyme monoamine oxidase (MAO). Redux works by preventing the uptake of serotonin by the platelets. If Redux is taken in conjunction with any drug that inhibits MAO activity, it can completely wipe out the body's ability to keep serotonin levels in check. Too much serotonin can harm blood vessels, particularly in the lungs, and can damage the valves of the heart. Redux labels, therefore, specifically warned against prescribing the drug to patients taking MAO-inhibitors.

In 1992, physicians began prescribing Redux in combination with an older drug, phentermine. Phentermine, a stimulant similar to amphetamine, tended to offset the sedating effects of Redux. And because the two drugs were not included in the same pill, the FDA did not require a separate study of the safety of prescribing them in tandem. Patients taking the combination reported a near total loss of appetite, and the resulting weight loss success stories were astounding. Reports of people dropping fifty or more pounds in a few months became commonplace.

And so the fen-phen craze was on. It was an American dream come true. No dieting, no exercise, no effort at all—just pop a couple of pills and you could lose all the weight you wanted. Word of mouth sent patients flocking to their doctors to ask for fen-phen, and by 1996 the two components of the combination had made the list of the top ten fastest-growing drugs in America.

Some of the more responsible physicians were reluctant to prescribe fen-phen, aware that the drug combination's safety had not been tested. But they were a small obstacle to patients determined to shed pounds effortlessly. Doctors at national weight loss chains like Nutri/System and Jenny Craig offered prescriptions. Fen-phen clinics began springing up all over, offering a cursory medical examination and a supply of pills for about $100 a month.

Then, in the summer of 1997, the "miracle" weight loss cure came crashing to earth when the FDA reported that eighty-two patients had developed heart-valve defects while on fen-phen, and another young woman had died of pulmonary hypertension. An article in *JAMA* reported that the drug combination can cause brain damage in laboratory animals. Within weeks the prescriptions for fen-phen plummeted, and that September the manufacturer of Redux voluntarily withdrew it from the market.

The problem was not just that this combination of drugs had been prescribed wholesale without adequate testing, but that the drug manufacturers and the medical community should have known all along of its potentially lethal consequences. The reason? Phentermine is an MAO-inhibitor. That fact had been known since the 1970s but was not mentioned in any of the common drug information materials such as the *Physicians' Desk Reference* or even on the medication's label. How did this happen? At the time phentermine was first released, its MAO-inhibiting effect was not known; and when it did become known, no one thought it was important enough to justify renegotiating the drug's FDA-approved label. So the information was largely ignored until 1997, when the effects of runaway blood serotonin levels in fen-phen patients finally were brought to the attention of the medical community.

American Home Products, the manufacturer of Pondimin and Redux, agreed in October 1999 to pay $3.75 billion to settle lawsuits from patients who claimed to have been injured by fen-phen.

Sadly, that wasn't the end of the fen-phen story. Even after the manufacturer recalled Pondimin and Redux, I still found doctors willing to prescribe the drugs and pharmacists willing to dispense them. In another television segment, I went to several diet clinics in Cleveland, Ohio (not the real location), pretending to be a patient who'd taken fen-phen in the past and was willing to do whatever it took to get my prescription for Pondimin refilled.

The first doctor I approached was offended by my request. He told me that he "would never have prescribed it to anyone to begin with, had I known about the heart-valve problems. That's not a side effect—that's like a death sentence."

Others were far less squeamish about my health.

At another clinic, the office manager—not a doctor—at first refused my requests and tried to convince me to switch to a different medication. I explained that I didn't want my prescriptions changed. Then I offered the man $1,200 cash. He reconsidered and told me that Pondimin was still available in a nearby state through the mail. But first I had to take a physical to make sure there wasn't anything wrong with me.

"We're not going to play Russian roulette with your heart," the man told me.

Yet the nurse who did my checkup failed to ask me about the fourteen-inch scar on my chest—a scar that was the result of open-heart surgery. Still, to get my prescription, I had to come back the next day to see the doctor.

On hidden camera, the doctor said, "There's no way I can prescribe it [Pondimin] in this state, I don't think. Let me talk to the guy out there and I'll be right back." After talking to the office manager, the doctor apparently changed his mind.

The doctor came back and told me, "Got it figured out. So what we're gonna do is, I'm gonna give you my little spiel, and I'll write the prescription here, which we will fax up to a pharmacy in Indiana (not the real location) and they will send the medicines to you."

Of course, the recall of Pondimin was nationwide, and the drug was no more legal in Indiana than in Ohio. The only difference was that the Indiana pharmacist was willing to run the risk of dispensing the drug.

After a short physical, the doctor wrote out a prescription for Pondimin, which would arrive via overnight shipping. Then the doctor told me, "There are side effects. I'm not gonna tell you about those. You're an intelligent guy. I'm sure you've read about it, seen it, and know what's going on."

I paid $50 for the Pondimin and went home. The next day, I returned to the clinic but my prescription hadn't arrived. Since the office manager was taking Pondimin himself, I asked him to give me his own personal prescription and take mine when it arrived.

"I can't do it," he replied. "That's against the law."

But he gave it to me anyway, jokingly commenting, "I didn't do that. You know, I don't know what happened to my pills. I, I didn't do anything."

Minutes later I revealed that I was a reporter and confronted the office manager on camera. He insisted that I'd taken the prescription out of his hands. When asked about the doctor in the clinic who gave me the prescription for Pondimin after the drug had been recalled, the office manager insisted that it had not been his decision.

I asked the man, "How would you feel if I developed a valvular disorder and died? Would that bother your conscience at all?"

He replied, "Yes, it would bother my conscience. But I'm not the one who manufactures the drug. I'm not the one that prescribes it. I'm just the one who sits here and works . . ."

"And sells it," I added.

He denied selling the drugs and suggested I take the matter up with the person who supplied the clinic's patients with Pondimin, the pharmacist in Indiana. So I did.

When I confronted the pharmacist with the office manager's assertions, the pharmacist's reaction was adamant. "That's a flat-out lie!" he told me.

I asked him, "Have you dispensed any Pondimin since you received the recall letter?"

He insisted he had not. I asked him again. "I don't believe so," he replied.

I asked the question yet again, using the name of the doctor who had written my prescription. The pharmacist replied, "I've filled prescriptions for him," then abruptly ended the interview, refusing to answer any more questions.

"Fat-Grabbers"

Another idea that works in theory far better than in reality are fat-grabbers, pills that supposedly allow you to eat fatty, high-calorie foods without gaining weight. According to promotional materials printed by one manufacturer, the substances in the pill bind with the fat in the meal and allow it to pass through the digestive system without being absorbed.

The principal ingredients in fat-grabbers are chitosan, a fiberlike substance made from the shells of shellfish, and psyllium husks, a plant fiber used in bulk laxatives like Metamucil. According to an August 16, 1999, story in USA Today, five Italian studies did in fact find that chitosan can contribute to weight loss. However, the subjects of these studies were already on low-calorie, low-fat diets and the weight loss contribution of chitosan was very small.

My own online search through the National Library of Medicine's Web site found over seven hundred research articles on chitosan, not one of which mentions it as a means of removing fat from the digestive system. I was able to find no scientific evidence to substantiate the claims that fat-grabbers really work.

Apparently I'm not the only one. Enforma Natural Products, which had marketed its product under the brand name Fat Trapper, ran television ads showing people eating foods like pizza and fried chicken, supposedly absorbing none of the enormous quantities of fat they contain. In a press release dated April 26, 2000, the FTC announced that Enforma Natural Products, Inc., had agreed to settle charges of false advertising by paying $10 million and agreeing to cease making deceptive claims about Fat Trapper. Previously, SlimAmerica, Inc., a Florida company that sold products similar to those of Enforma, had been fined over $8 million in consumer redress after the FTC filed suit against them for false and misleading advertising. Their ads claimed their "Super-Formula" could "blast" up to forty-nine pounds off in only twenty-nine days without the need to diet and exercise. Such settlements don't constitute any admission of legal violation by the defendants, however.

"Exercise Pills"

If the claims of the fat-grabbers seem far-fetched, how about a pill that gives you the benefits of an exercise program without moving a muscle? According to Enforma Natural Products, their Exercise In a Bottle product would allow you to burn more calories while standing still.

Again, the claims start with a small shred of truth. The principal ingredient of Exercise In a Bottle is calcium pyruvate. A 1999 study published in the *International Journal of Sport Nutrition* found that football players who took a combination of creatine monohydrate and calcium pyruvate while training did show an increase in lean body mass and athletic performance over those who did not take the supplements. However, the supplements only worked when taken in addition to, not instead of, a vigorous exercise program. Further, the study found that pyruvate supplementation by itself was ineffective.

There is absolutely no evidence to show that a bottle of pills can substitute for a regular exercise program. The FTC concurred, and Enforma agreed to stop making such claims as a part of its $10 million deceptive advertising settlement (discussed earlier)

"Fat-Storage Blockers"

Another entertaining weight loss idea is for a pill that blocks the body from storing fat. That's the claim made by those who tout herbal weight-loss products containing extracts of the bitter orange, *Garcinia cambogia*.

Garcinia does indeed contain an enzyme that could, in theory anyway, inhibit the body's ability to create and store fat. To test whether it actually works in this way, doctors at Columbia University's Obesity Research Center conducted a carefully controlled study on a group of overweight adults enrolled in a weight loss program. The results, reported in *JAMA,* were disappointing, to say the least. It was found that *Garcinia* supplementation was no more effective than a placebo in helping the study participants lose weight.

Acupressure

Some patients have reported the successful use of acupuncture and its less "needling" alternative—acupressure—in the treatment of obesity. The idea is that by stimulating certain nerves you can curb the appetite.

A Florida company took this concept another step further in developing the Acu-Stop 2000, a plastic earpiece that supposedly stimulated the nerve endings in a way that produced a feeling of fullness in the stomach. These devices, which cost an estimated 14 cents each to produce, were marketed for $39.95, plus shipping and handling.

In 1995, the FDA's health fraud investigators cracked down on the distributors of Acu-Stop 2000 and seized the company's entire inventory, which had a retail value of over half a million dollars. Most of these scam devices were incinerated, but Bob McCoy at the Museum of Questionable Medical Devices sent me a few. As a part of a *Hard Copy* TV segment, I decided to see for myself just how easy it was to con people with this improbable device. Wearing a white smock with a stethoscope around my neck, I set up a sales booth in a mall. From my booth I hawked the Acu-Stop 2000 as a fast, safe, and effective way to lose weight and keep it off. All buyers had to do was wear the device twice a day—three minutes in the morning and three minutes before bed at night. I even told them that it was FDA-approved.

I had no trouble finding people who were so desperate to lose weight they would plunk down $40 for a worthless plastic earpiece. I told one young long-haired brunette, "We have people who have lost twenty pounds in one month."

The woman rolled her eyes and opened her mouth in astonishment. Then she looked over at her friend. "Hey, if I want to lose ten pounds. . . ."

I reassured her that if it didn't work for her, the device came with a money-back guarantee. After she'd handed over two $20 bills, I showed her a letter from the Department of Health and Human Services explaining that the FDA and U.S. Marshals in Florida had seized 19,000 of the devices because they were a sham. Then she snatched back her money out of my hands. When I showed the letter to another woman who'd bought an Acu-Stop 2000, she asked me if she was under arrest!

Why were so many people willing to plunk down hard-earned cash for a bogus device? As one senior citizen who fell for the scam put it, most were "willing to try anything if it would help."

The people who invented the Acu-Stop 2000 must have been aware of the appeal of their phony device to desperate people. In the true spirit of MediScam entrepreneurialism, the company also advertised an Acu-Stop 3000—with a slightly different twist: This device was supposed to help in the cessation of smoking.

CHELATION THERAPY

Chelation is actually a legitimate clinical therapy that has been put to illegitimate use by certain elements of the medical community. This therapy consists of infusing patients with a solution of the chemical ethylenediaminetetraacetic acid (EDTA). (How's that for a spelling bee tie breaker?) The term "chelate" comes from the Greek word *chele*, or "claw," and refers to the clawlike structure of the EDTA molecule that binds to certain metallic ions dissolved in water. Shortly after EDTA was first synthesized in the 1930s, it was found it could be used successfully to remove toxic heavy metals such as lead from the human bloodstream. EDTA chelation is still recognized by the mainstream medical community as a valid therapy for heavy-metal poisoning.

Early on, some scientists had postulated that because EDTA also binds calcium, it might be useful in softening the calcified deposits lining the blood vessels of patients suffering from arteriosclerosis. And in 1956, three doctors chelating patients who suffered from one form of hardening of the arteries reported their patients had reported a decrease of symptoms after treatment with EDTA.

Since that time an entire industry has developed around using chelation therapy as an alternative to surgery in the treatment of circulatory diseases. Chelation proponents include members of the *American College for Advancement in Medicine* (ACAM), a professional organization which has not only promoted the widespread use of chelation therapy but produces its own publications, including the *American Journal of Advancement of Medicine*. Neither ACAM nor its publications, however, are recognized by the mainstream medical and scientific communities.

The problem is that the only truly scientific studies of chelation therapy show that it is useless in treating anything other than heavy-metal poisoning. And a true "double-blind" study—comparing patients who have actually been chelated with those who have not—has never been performed. Why? The drug companies aren't going to fund such a study because EDTA is a cheap generic chemical that cannot be patented; therefore the drug companies have no financial incentive to investigate its clinical uses.

Nor is ACAM likely to fund such a study. Patients undergoing chelation therapy typically undergo around thirty or so treatments, each costing $75 to $125. The doctors' only direct expenses are for a saline-infusion bag and a few cents for the EDTA, so the profit margin is huge. And because only a handful of physicians nationwide offer chelation therapy (ACAM has fewer than one thousand members in the U.S.), and the number of patients seeking the treatment is so large (an estimated 300,000 to 500,000 patients have already undergone it), chelation doctors are often swamped with business. If ACAM *were* to prove that chelation is a safe and effective alternative to coronary bypass surgery, the treatment would become routine for doctors everywhere. And that, of course, would severely erode the income base of ACAM's membership.

However, ACAM may have an incentive to conduct such studies. The FTC recently concluded that, in truth and in fact, scientific studies do not prove that EDTA chelation therapy is an effective treatment for arteriosclerosis. ACAM recently agreed to settle a case brought against it by the government agency by agreeing that it would stop advertising chelation therapy as safe and effective against arteriosclerosis.

Thus, in the case of chelation therapy, we have a treatment based on incomplete science. And because no one has an economic incentive to actually prove or disprove its clinical effectiveness, the science behind the therapy is likely to remain incomplete. So the MediScam continues, and even grows in complexity. Because insurance companies will pay for chelation therapy when used to treat heavy-metal poisoning but not other conditions, it's not unusual for a chelation therapy doctor to falsely diagnose such poisoning in order to get insurance coverage. Although the insurance companies are cracking down on this practice, it still continues.

SCIENCE AND INFORMED CONSENT

With legitimate physicians sometimes getting—and giving—scientifically inappropriate advice, it may seem that even the most intelligent and wary patient doesn't stand a chance anymore. Fortunately, there are protections. Unfortunately, you may actually have to be injured by a scientifically unsound treatment before you can use them.

An important legal protection is your right to give informed consent to treatment. The basic principle of informed consent is that, *after having been properly educated by the practitioner* about the risks and benefits of the proposed treatment, and about the viable treatment options, including the option of no treatment, the patient has the right to choose freely whether to submit to treatment. The key phrase here is the one in italics. Unless the physician or other practitioner has provided the patient with scientifically valid, accurate information about the treatment, a state of informed consent does not exist. That means that the practitioner, not the patient, is legally liable for any bad outcome, even if the patient was warned that the bad outcome was possible. Under these circumstances, even a signed consent form becomes little more than a worthless scrap of paper.

The bottom line is this: Under the law there is no such thing as informed consent to quackery. "Experimental" treatments, like any others, must have a valid scientific rationale. If you are injured in any way because you relied on unsound or bogus scientific claims to justify a medical treatment, you can and should take the offender to court.

But it's also a good idea for patients to educate and protect themselves. Organizations like the American Heart Association, the American Cancer Society, and other long-standing, legitimate advocacy groups provide abundant patient education materials. They also provide direction to patients who are trying to decide if a proposed "experimental" treatment is legitimate or just another scam.

chapter 7

Marketing MediScams

Fraud as a Multimedia Event

HOW CAN YOU TELL the bogus products from the legitimate ones? Usually, by the way they are marketed. Once you understand how they work, it's usually fairly easy to recognize a scam. Let me give a few examples to show you what I mean.

FRAUD BY MAIL

From 1988 through 1993 Kenneth Thiefault, a self-proclaimed scientist and clinical researcher (who was later found to have no scientific background), used the U.S. mail extensively to tout ozone as a cure-all for almost every known disease: cancer, herpes, AIDS, hepatitis, gangrene—to name a few. And for $4,800, he would sell you an ozone-generating machine that you could use to cure yourself of incurable diseases right in the comfort of your own home. Not only that, his apparatus came with attachments you could use to bathe in an ozone-saturated body bag, or even to blow ozone directly up your anus.

Ozone, a gas whose molecules contain three atoms of oxygen instead of the normal two present in the oxygen we breathe, is a powerful oxidizer that does, indeed, kill germs. So does laundry bleach. And to say that saturating yourself with ozone will cure diseases is equivalent to saying that bathing in bleach will also cure diseases. But then, logic and MediScams rarely go well together.

The FDA repeatedly warned Thiefault he was marketing an unapproved medical device, and that this was illegal. In order to get FDA approval, he had to submit data showing that his devices were both safe and clinically effective in living up to the claims he made about them. Thiefault never produced such data.

By 1993 the FDA's Office of Criminal Investigations had enough evidence to obtain a search warrant and raid Thiefault's home. The investigation, complemented by an IRS investigation into unpaid back taxes, led to a seven-count indictment against Thiefault and his wife, Mardel Barber. After a two-week trial, they were found guilty of mail fraud, wire fraud, and distribution of an unapproved medical device. Thiefault was sentenced to six and a half years in prison, fined $100,000, and ordered to pay $14,400 in restitution. Barber got almost three years in prison and was fined $60,000. Both were also banned from dealing in securities, telemarketing, direct mailings, and nationwide advertising.

How many times have you received a postcard, letter, or brochure in the mail touting some new medical product or device? If you have a medical condition and have ordered relevant medical supplies or information by phone or mail, chances are you've made someone's targeted mailing list—so, small wonder you receive a brochure for an arthritis cure when you've got arthritis. The problem, of course, is separating the MediScams from the legitimate treatments. Although the U.S. Postal Service does its best to rout out the fraudulent offers, often it takes weeks or months—and a lot of consumer complaints—to put a stop to them.

Mail fraud is "a criminal scheme where the postal system is used to obtain money or anything of value from a victim by offering a product, service, or investment opportunity that does not live up to its claims." The Mail Fraud Statute (Title 18, United States Code, Section 1341), enacted in 1872, is the nation's oldest federal consumer-protection law. Recently, the U.S. Postal Service changed private mailbox identification procedures to protect private businesses that accept customers' mail from the post office, hold it in a private mailbox, or redirect it to a new address. This change was in response to concerns that private mailboxes were being used to shield illegal activities and to illegally reroute goods and services.

The mail system has been in common use for over 150 years. And until private delivery companies came into being, the mail system was the only means to send a package from point A to point B. Besides being marketed by mail through brochures and postcards, many bogus products have been and still are sent through the U.S. Postal Service. And that makes the sender vulnerable to prosecution under the mail fraud statutes.

If you observe a bogus promotion being offered through the mails, you should file a Mail Fraud Report with the U.S. Postal Inspection Service. They have a special category for "Medical Quackery," which includes the subcategories of "Weight Loss," "AIDS Cure," "Cancer Cure," and "Sexual Aid." The U.S. Postal Inspection Service's Web site at http:/www.usps.gov/postalinspectors has valuable information on what to look for, how to prevent being taken by a quack cure, and other information about mail fraud.

FRAUD BY PHONE

Chapter 2 of this book presents a brief discussion of a device known as the "Dynamizer" and its historical place in the annals of medical quackery devices. What's even more fascinating is that the Dynamizer's inventor and promoter, Albert Abrams, M.D., has the dubious distinction of being one of the earliest MediScammers to use the telephone to promote medical quackery. And while most of the quacks we've discussed so far were either bogus or incompetent physicians, Albert Abrams was neither.

Albert Abrams was a distinguished and well-respected physician with impressive credentials that included doctorates in both medicine and law. Born in 1863, he earned his medical degree while still a teenager at the University of Heidelberg. He later became the chief pathologist at what would become the Stanford University School of Medicine. He wrote hundreds of medical articles in prestigious medical journals, and physicians worldwide sought Abrams' professional counsel. By the early 1900s he had become one of the most respected neurologists (doctors who treat diseases of the nervous system) in America. Unfortunately, the recognition and financial remuneration were not enough for him, and Abrams often told colleagues and friends that he sought to be a prophet among men.

When he published a book on "spondylotherapy," his version of chiropractic and osteopathy (which were looked upon as cults by traditional medicine) in 1910, his peers started viewing him with suspicion. Soon, Abrams was giving clinical courses on spondylotherapy in various parts of the country for $50. Eventually, he offered a four-week course in San Francisco for $200. By 1916 he had begun creating his latest theory, which culminated in Abrams' most famous invention, the "Dynamizer." With its fine-finished walnut case, it looked more like a piece of furniture with dials and lights than a medical device.

According to Abrams' new theory, which came to be called the Electronic Reactions of Abrams, or "ERA," electrons were the basis of life. He believed that the human body transmits electronic vibrations. As such, every disease had a telltale electronic signature. Abrams reasoned that one could cure a disease by transmitting its electronic vibratory rate back at it.

Using a drop of blood from the patient, the Dynamizer was able to "read" the patient's ERA. Connected to the Dynamizer by head gear was a healthy individual who, while facing west, would react to the diseased vibrations. The doctor could detect the disease and its specific location by thumping the abdomen of the healthy person.

Not only could the doctor diagnose syphilis, diabetes, cancer, tuberculosis, and dozens of other maladies using the Dynamizer, Abrams bragged he could tell a patient's age, sex, religion, and whether he played the ponies. If a drop of blood wasn't available, a hair or writing sample would work just as well. Abrams even claimed to have diagnosed the diseases of individuals who died long ago.

Doctors from around the world attended Abrams' special workshops in San Francisco to learn about and be trained on the hottest new diagnostic instrument in medical history. Abrams told his receptive audiences that all other diagnostic instruments were archaic and obsolete. After all, he would argue convincingly, his Dynamizer was noninvasive, painless, and accurate 100 percent of the time. This truly was a medical miracle.

In 1920 Abrams introduced another new device, this one called the Oscilloclast. This instrument had a magnet to polarize blood samples, then would read the "vibratory rate" and diagnose diseases from the sample. Not only that, but it would cure the patient by bombarding him with vibrations that "canceled out" the vibrations from the disease.

To top off Abram's remarkable claims, he said the patient could even send a blood sample through the mail or phone it in to one of his many telemarketing operators. The operators were supposedly trained to read the vibratory rate of the blood sample through the phone line for a mere $5!

Attendees of Abrams' workshop could lease the machine by putting up a $200 to $250 deposit (depending on whether it was wired for direct or alternating current) and paying a usage charge of $5 per week (or per month—accounts vary).

Those who signed the contracts were admonished never to look inside Abrams' equipment, since breaking the seal would permanently damage the apparatus. The attendees, in turn, returned home and charged their patients as much as $200 per reading.

Everyone was making a fortune—the doctors who used the machine were raking in up to $2,000 per week. And Abrams, of course, was becoming incredibly wealthy. An article by the Museum of Medical Quackery recounts the testimonial of one of Abrams' disciples published in Abrams' *Physico-Clinical Medicine* and quoted in the *Journal of the American Medical Association* on March 25, 1922:

The Oscilloclast has doubled my business.

—*S. King, M.D. (Pennsylvania)*

Other testimonials glowingly touted successful results on patients:

Woman. Age 52—Diagnosis of acquired syphilis made by one of our most eminent clinicians . . . Abrams test showed tuberculosis of the apex of the right lung. No syphilis. Fourteen treatments with the Oscilloclast at 5. Patient gained fourteen pounds in three weeks. Now in perfect health.

Cancer of the uterus. Inoperable. Severe uterine hemorrhages. Electrode of Oscilloclast to cervix and hemorrhage ceased after second treatment. After 14 treatments the patient was declared well. Another case of the same character was followed by equally good results.

Is it little wonder that his followers loved him so much? Nobody wanted to think about the consequences of Abrams' being a fraud. Nobody except the AMA and *Scientific American* magazine.

The AMA's position regarding Abrams' claims was that he was possibly the biggest quack of the twentieth century. *JAMA* recounted that the abilities of ERA practitioners to diagnose disease had been put to the test when blood samples sent through the mail turned out to be those of a male guinea pig, who was diagnosed with a *Streptococcus* infection of the left fallopian tube, and a rooster, who was diagnosed with venereal disease. The AMA magazine *Hygeia* (which became *Today's Health)* called Abrams "the most finished medical charlatan of our time," according to author Ken Raines.

In December 1923 *Scientific American* put together a committee of physicians to determine whether or not Abrams' machines worked. The committee was formed after an elderly man who had been diagnosed with cancer died a month after he had supposedly been cured by treatment with one of Abrams' machines. Also clamoring for a scientific test of the machines were hundreds of doctors from around the world who did not use the Dynamizer or the Oscilloclast. These physicians complained they were losing patients to doctors who did use the machines, and that many of those patients were probably dying as a result of having been misdiagnosed and given inappropriate medical treatment.

To test Abrams' equipment, an ERA practitioner in New York City was asked to analyze the contents of six vials. He was then asked to diagnose the disease based upon the readings. When he failed during the first trial, the doctor found the cause of his unsuccessful diagnoses: There was a touch of red on each of the vial's labels, which was fatal to the accuracy of the electronic reactions. There was also handwriting on the labels, which carried electronic emissions from the writer. Even after the committee had new labels with typed numbers attached according to the doctor's specifications, subsequent tests produced other diagnoses that were completely wrong. The doctor misdiagnosed all six. Additional tests by other ERA practitioners were equally unsuccessful. *Scientific American* concluded,

> This committee finds that the claims advanced on behalf of the electronic reaction of Abrams, and of electronic practice in general, are not substantiated; and it is our belief that they have no basis in fact. In our opinion the so-called electronic treatments are without value.

Abrams accused the committee of ignorance and claimed that he was being victimized. However, the resulting press coverage was devastating for the doctors who used the machines, and Abrams never conducted tests to prove the efficacy of his inventions. When one of his machines was opened it was found to contain nothing more than a few meaningless dials and electrical gadgets wired together—nothing that could even remotely hope to live up to the diagnostic and curative claims made by Abrams.

Abrams died at age fifty-five of pneumonia in an Arkansas motel room the night before he was to testify in a mail fraud case. It is not known how many people were diagnosed and treated with Abrams' machines. Nor will we ever know how many died or suffered needlessly because they failed to seek legitimate medical treatment. What we do know is that Albert Abrams will be remembered as one of the most successful—and despicable—quacks in the annals of medical history.

Telemarketing is a powerful medium for selling bogus cures and products. A salesperson, perhaps already aware of your need of a miracle cure, might prey on your vulnerability by promising a cure or your money back. It's easy—you just give them a credit card number, and the answer to all your problems is delivered to your doorstep a few days later. It's private—no one needs to know if you bought something by phone. And telemarketers can be persuasive, using medical jargon that may sound good but mean nothing. Even patients who are suspicious can sometimes be sold. After all, it's only money, and who can resist the allure of a quick cure?

Telemarketing fraud, one of the most pervasive and problematic forms of white-collar crime, is being actively fought through a consumer-education initiative called kNOw FRAUD. The government estimates that Americans, more than half over the age of fifty, are bilked out of $40 billion annually from illegal telemarketing schemes. kNOw FRAUD is a program designed to educate people about fraud and how to spot it, as well as provide an easy way to report fraud. The program has been launched by the U.S. Postal Inspection Service, the American Association of Retired Persons, the Council of Better Business Bureaus, the Department of Justice, the FBI, the FTC, the National Association of Attorneys General, and the Securities and Exchange Commission. President Bill Clinton, Andy Griffith, and I produced public service announcements to launch the program. Best of all, the entire cost for kNOw FRAUD was paid with fines levied against a fraudulent telemarketing company. Now *that's* justice!

INFOMERCIALS—
Making Advertising Look Like Entertainment

It's late at night and you're flipping channels when you come across what appears to be a talk show. The host sits behind his desk, appearing thoroughly fascinated as his guest, Kevin Trudeau, explains that his Mega

Memory System can help anyone achieve a photographic memory. Guaranteed to work for even the mentally handicapped, the techniques increase recall ability from 15 to 90 percent in just five days, he explains. Sounds far-fetched, but the inventor wouldn't be invited on this talk show if it didn't work, right? You settle back and listen intently, realizing that the Mega Memory System just might be the answer to your "senior moments." As you start to wonder how you can get your hands on his revolutionary new system, there's a commercial break and—aren't you lucky!—the commercial just happens to be for Trudeau's product.

Of course, what neither the host nor his guest is telling you is that the entire program, including the fake talk-show format, is nothing more than a staged commercial. Nor are they telling you that Trudeau and all the other guests appearing on this "talk show" have paid for the privilege of being there in order to hawk their wares. And most importantly of all, they're certainly not telling you that the claims about their products—which range from "Eden's Secret Nature's Purifying System" (an herbal colon cleanser which is supposed to enhance the overall integrity of your body) to Jacqueline Sable's "Hair Farming System" (touted to be more effective than Minoxidil in fighting baldness)—are all bogus according to the FTC.

But wait, there's more. In January 1998 Trudeau and eight other marketers who hawked their products using false claims on ersatz talk-show infomercials were charged by the FTC with false advertising. The defendants agreed to pay $1.1 million to settle the claims. Kevin Trudeau was ordered to set up a $500,000 escrow account to be used in the future should he commit similar violations. All of the defendants settled the charges by agreeing to cease making false and misleading claims about their products. Sable, who settled separately, is barred for life from selling any product claiming to treat or prevent baldness. Consent agreements are for settlement purposes only and do not constitute admissions of law violations.

"Infomercials," commercials adapted to the length and general formatting of traditional entertainment programming, are the electronic age's answer to the traveling medicine show. They got their initial boost in 1984 when the Federal Communications Commission (FCC) dropped regulations regarding the maximum amount of commercial time local stations could air. From the stations' standpoint, infomercials were a godsend. Before infomercials, a station would have to buy programming to fill those little-watched hours between midnight and six A.M., then face the onerous task of selling commercials to sponsor the shows. But with infomercials, the sponsor provided entertainment and sponsorship all in one. And the results are profitable for station and sponsor alike. In big-city markets, a half-hour infomercial can bring the station between $5,000 and $20,000 per screening, with very little cost or effort to the station. And the profit on the sponsor's side can be breathtaking. To give just one example, a half-hour infomercial about a hand mixer from Kitchenmate cost just $125,000 to make, yet brought in over $55 million in sales.

How can you tell if it's an infomercial? The FCC requires that stations disclose who's paying for an infomercial at its beginning or its end. The best way to identify an infomercial is that the commercials will cover the same material as the program content. Another giveaway is if the program gives information about ordering the product. Authentic talk shows keep program content and commercials strictly separated.

There's nothing illegal about using an infomercial to advertise products. If you're watching an infomercial, remember that it's nothing more than an extended advertisement, and the claims made during the program should be evaluated accordingly. When you watch a one-minute standard commercial, you know better than to take all its claims too seriously. While not all infomercials offer bogus merchandise, it's important to be cautious. Ask yourself why, if the product is as good as its promoters claim, do they need an entire half hour to sell it? There may be a legitimate reason. But don't be suckered into thinking that they couldn't make such claims on TV if they weren't true. People can, and do, lie to you—as much on infomercials as they do in any other medium. While it's true that the FTC tries to keep infomercials honest, it may take months for the agency to act. In the meantime, thousands of customers can be duped by the MediScammers producing the infomercial.

ENDORSEMENTS AND TESTIMONIALS

Celebrity endorsements are a tried-and-true method of selling goods and services, and you'll see celebrities flogging every manner of product on every medium in which advertising appears. But you have to ask yourself, "So what if my favorite celebrity endorses this product? Does he or she know any more about it than anyone else?" Take the case of the soap- opera star who opened his 1980s TV ads for pain relievers with the line, "I'm not a doctor, but I play one on TV." By what stretch of the imagination would playing a doctor on TV make him an expert on med-ications? And even if his acting job *did* bestow such knowledge, we must not lose sight of the fact celebrities are *paid* for endorsing products. The mere fact that someone collects a paycheck from a company certainly doesn't give him any knowledge or insight into the company's products.

Another favored advertising gimmick, especially among Medi-Scammers, is the patient's endorsement. As we'll see in chapter 10 about placebos, virtually any product or service, no matter how useless, will have its proponents, and those proponents will offer glowing testimonials. But so what? Remember, the company certainly isn't going to advertise comments from *dis*satisfied customers which may far outnumber those who speak favorably about its products. And how do you even know that the testimonials are real in the first place? Consider the following Web site testimonial for an herbal breast-enlargement product called Grobust:

I just recently started on Grobust and I have had astonishing results—one-half inch in the first 10 days. After 3 months I have grown 2 inches!

—J. T. (Ivins, Utah)

Unless you're willing to go through the phone book and contact women in Ivins, Utah, with the initials J. T., there's simply no way to determine if this testimonial is even real, let alone whether it accurately reflects the kind of results you might expect if you were to take this product yourself.

MULTILEVEL MARKETING—
Recruiting Friends and Family to Become MediScammers

While most multilevel marketing (MLM) companies sell legitimate products and offer certain economic advantages to the consumer in bypassing retail distribution costs, others are run by con artists who cannot resist the temptation of recruiting thousands of distributors to sell their bogus products.

MLM firms can be an ideal vehicle for MediScammers to sell their snake oil. Unscrupulous scammers feed half-truths and mistruths to prospective distributors in order to convince them to sign up and get rich. The new distributors, in turn, repeat the deceptions in order to sign up friends, family, and co-workers. After all, it's a lot easier to believe your next-door neighbor's claims about these miraculous new products than the pitch of some fast-talking barker on a TV infomercial. And so the virus spreads, with very little work or advertising by the company. What could be easier—or more profitable for the company?

But beware of any claims about so-called miracle products. Entrepreneurial upstarts trying to build their own downlines (distributors under them from whom they collect a commission on sales) may be tempted to exaggerate a product's usefulness in order to increase sales. When distributors attend regional or national meetings, they hear success story after success story about fellow distributors who live in mansions, drive expensive sports cars, and entertain on their own yachts. Of course, what the company fails to point out is that these success stories are more likely to come from recruiting more distributors than from selling superior products.

Case in point—the ads started out like this: "The problem: Johnny isn't staying up with the rest of the children, he's getting into fights at recess and he's just not listening." The MLM company New Vision had the solution.

"God's Recipe," a natural health product comprised of three dietary supplements, claimed it was a cure for Attention Deficit Disorder (ADD) or Attention Deficit/Hyperactivity Disorder (ADHD), and its ads stated it was making a huge difference in the lives of thousands of children. An FTC press release stated this was the first case the FTC had investigated involving ADD/ADHD, a disorder that affects some 2.5 million American kids.

In 1999 the FTC ordered New Vision International, Inc., to stop making claims that its products could cure, prevent, treat, or mitigate ADD, ADHD, or their symptoms, or that their products were effective alternative treatments for Ritalin, unless they had reliable scientific evidence of these claims. The firm was told it must keep a watchful eye over the claims its distributors make, too, by instituting a program where independent distributors must submit all advertising for pre-approval. Should an independent distributor fail to do so, or make representations about products that couldn't be backed up with scientific evidence, the distributor could be suspended or terminated. Although New Vision and its principles agreed to settle the FTC charges, such an agreement does not constitute an admission of a law violation.

Nu Skin International, Inc., another MLM company, paid $1.5 million to settle charges it made unsubstantiated claims on five of its products that supposedly reduced fat, increased metabolism, and built muscle, according to the FTC. The FTC alleged that Nu Skin couldn't substantiate its claims, therefore violating a 1994 FTC order requiring them to have competent and reliable evidence for claims about their products. Nu Skin agreed to abide by the 1994 order in the future. Consent decrees have the force of law when signed by a judge, but are for settlement purposes only. They do not constitute an admission by the defendant of a law violation.

THE NEWEST MEDIUM—The Internet

The Internet has become a virtual shopping mall for bogus products. One stunning example is the "Androstenone Pheromone Concentrate" from Amazing Products, Inc. Imagine getting an e-mail whose subject line reads: "Attract Women Now!!!" If you read the text, the sales pitch goes on to state that Androstenone Pheromone Concentrate "unblocks all restraints and unleashes her raw animal sex drive. Scientists have isolated the natural human male Pheromone attractants and they are NOW available to YOU, legally, in the U.S.!" To lend credence to its claims, the company stated that its product had been featured on the TV shows *Hard Copy, 20/20,* and *Dateline NBC,* and in magazines such as *Penthouse, Playboy, Vogue, Omni, Discovery*, numerous medical journals, and in newspapers such as the *New York Times* and the *Los Angeles Times.*

The U.S. Postal Inspection Service's case against Dennis P. Wilkie, doing business as Amazing Products, Inc., resulted in an agreement containing a consent order to cease and desist. In that order Wilkie agreed to stop claiming, or even implying, that his Androstenone Pheromone Concentrate causes women to become sexually attracted to the male who uses it.

A Bogus HIV Test

For consumers who purchased the Lei-Home Access HIV Test or Personal HIV Test Kit, the first hint that something was wrong should have come when they looked at the kit. It came in a plain white cardboard box with a computer-generated label. The next clue came when the box was opened. Inside was a card with an opened Band-Aid, a stylus, and another Band-Aid. The directions were to prick your finger, put a drop of blood on the open Band-Aid, then mail the card and Band-Aid back to the lab where it would be tested. The other Band-Aid was to cover the pinprick.

The test kit, which retailed for around $40, was sold over the Internet and also marketed to pharmacies over the phone. An investigation into the operation was launched when the FDA's Center for Biologics Evaluation and Research, which regulates HIV home sample-collection kits, received complaints from the industry about an unapproved test kit.

Subsequent inquiries revealed that the tests were marketed by Lawrence Greene of Los Banos, California. Further investigation revealed that his tests were not only unapproved, they were downright bogus. Greene had no laboratory facilities for testing the blood samples, and simply assigned them a random "positive" or "negative" result. The FDA immediately moved to shut down the operation. All remaining test kits were seized and the FDA contacted all those customers who had already received their "results" from Greene and advised them to be re-tested by a legitimate laboratory immediately. They also posted notices on the doors of the pharmacies where the kits had been sold.

In December 1997 Greene was indicted on multiple counts of mail fraud and wire fraud and jailed without bail. At trial the prosecution stressed the human impact of Greene's scam. Some patients who had been given bogus positive results had suffered the anguish of falsely believing that they were HIV-positive. Others who had been given bogus negative results may well have gone on to infect others, acting on the belief that they were not carrying the virus. The judge, impressed with the human toll Greene took on innocent lives, sentenced him to five years and three months in prison—a more severe punishment than is usual for fraud cases. Greene also has the dubious distinction of being the first person to be convicted for an FDA-prosecuted Internet fraud case.

Recruiting for a Pseudomedical Therapy

The Internet has heavily impacted the marketing of products—*any* product. For example, promoters of BioResonance Therapy, or BRT (discussed in chapter 2 as a variation of "Electroacupuncture according to Voll," or EAV) use e-mail, discussion groups, and a Web site to sell "the most effective new development for the natural elimination of tumors and their underlying causes yet discovered." Not only are they seeking 240 cancer patients to participate in their therapy for an estimated $14,000 ($9,000 for the six-week treatment, plus travel and lodging in Tijuana, Mexico, for an additional $5,000), but they offer a training program to become a certified BRT therapist at a cost of $100 per day for eighteen days. A medical researcher in Germany, Roland Ziegler, writes that testing of BRT devices by several groups of physicians and technicians showed it was a simple device with a computer processor in it and something that made the lights blink. He also writes that in September 1995, a federal German advisory board of physicians labeled "all kinds of bioresonance as totally ineffective pseudomedical treatment."

Why are people so vulnerable to products sold on the Internet? Internet experts would say it's because Americans are susceptible to a gullibility which weakens their ability to question what they read on e-mail, and compels them to e-mail copies to their family and friends. Psychologists and sociologists believe that because e-mail is new, people trust it.

Scott Reents, an analyst with Cyber Dialogue, a market research company that tracks the Internet, estimates that in 1998 22.3 million adults in the U.S. sought health care information from the Internet, which contains an estimated 15,000 to 17,000 health care Web sites. About four hundred of these sites were identified as containing questionable promotions during the 1997 and 1998 "health claims surf days," in which FTC investigators and public-health advocates from twenty-five countries identified Web sites that made false or deceptive advertising claims for products or services claiming to cure, treat, or prevent AIDS, arthritis, cancer, diabetes, heart disease, and MS.

After the sweep, four cases were identified where respondents were forced to stop making deceptive and unsubstantiated claims on their Web sites. The products or devices involved included magnetic-therapy devices that claimed to be effective in treating cancer, HIV, high blood pressure, arthritis, and other conditions, a fatty acid from beef tallow that claimed to cure most forms of arthritis, and capsules of shark cartilage and a liquid containing Cat's Claw (a Peruvian plant derivative) that were "scientifically proven" treatments for cancer, HIV/AIDS, and arthritis. None of the four companies admitted wrongdoing.

The FTC sent warnings to other companies with dubious products, reminding them that laws against deceptive advertising also applied to the Internet. Two months after this warning the FTC did a follow-up check on a representative sample of sixty-four sites. Of these, 72 percent were operating as usual, about 13 percent had dropped unsubstantiated claims or disappeared from the Internet, 10 percent had made other changes, and 5 percent couldn't be found. By 1998 the number of sites that had dropped their unsubstantiated claims had risen to 28 percent.

RECOGNIZING AND AVOIDING MEDICAL QUACKERY

We must never forget that advertisers can, and do, lie to us in *every* medium. The mere fact that a product is advertised in a flyer, or a magazine, on TV, over the Internet, or distributed by a trusted friend does not mean that the claims made about that product are valid.

No matter how a bogus treatment or product is marketed, the sales pitch from MediScammers is usually the same. Since the medical problems most commonly targeted by scam artists are serious diseases such as cancer, HIV and AIDS, and arthritis, it's easy to let desperation take control. Don't waste your time and money on worthless treatments. Talk to a health care professional and do your own research. Again, investigate the resources in the back of this book for guidance.

chapter 8

What on Earth?

Turning the Planet into Scam Cures

WHAT WOULDN'T ANY OF us give for a panacea, a universal remedy that would cure every ailment—or at least most of them—known to man and make you younger in the process? According to at least one self-described scientist, such a panacea actually does exist, one that will cure about 150 diseases including cancer, heart disease, diabetes, and arthritis. And what is this magic elixir? Calcium carbonate, the building-block of everything from eggshells to limestone to human bones. This isn't the same old generic calcium carbonate we find in some antacid tablets or even in blackboard chalk. Where's the money to be made in that? No, his panacea comes in the form of crushed coral, the skeletons of small ocean-dwelling animals that make up tropical reefs.

As with many MediScams, the promoter's contentions begin with legitimate but outdated scientific research. The theories are based on the work of German physician and two-time Nobel Laureate Otto Warburg who, seventy-five years ago, discovered that cancer cells exhibited a drop in pH, thus becoming more acidic. Warburg's part-time associate, the late Canadian-born physician Carl J. Reich, would carry this finding to the absurd extreme that a person's state of health was directly correlated to the pH of the bodily fluids.

This correlation was so clear-cut, Reich insisted, one could detect the presence or absence of disease simply by applying litmus paper to the saliva. If the saliva tested alkaline, the person was healthy; and if it tested acidic, the person was diseased. And the nonsense didn't stop there. The diseased person could be restored to health, Reich maintained, simply by bringing the bodily fluids back to an alkaline pH—by feeding the person calcium carbonate. The medical community eventually caught up with Reich and he was stripped of his Canadian and California medical licenses in 1987. Still, he continued to promote his outlandish ideas until his death a few years later.

Today, these theories continue to be promoted. One company says that the coral used in its products comes from the reefs off the Japanese island of Okinawa. Why Okinawa? Because there are 3 million people on Okinawa (a revelation that must come as a shock to the local census-takers, who record only 1.3 million), and the population has an average life span of 106 years (another shock for census-takers, who record life expectancies of age seventy-seven for men and eighty-five for women). But his most startling revelation is that the people of Okinawa are virtually cancer-free. One must wonder why Japan's National Cancer Center Research Institute classifies Okinawa as a "high-risk" area for developing lung cancer. But then, why let the facts get in the way of a good sales pitch?

To share in the Okinawans' remarkable legacy, all one needs do is to purchase sachets of crushed Okinawan coral for around $1 each, then dissolve each sachet in one or two quarts of water and drink it. The claims continue: without providing any verification whatever, it seems that 100 percent of one vendor's coral calcium is absorbed by the body, compared with only about 5 percent absorption for all other forms of calcium. And the claims don't stop there. Why, you can even spray the coral calcium solution on plants to rid them of bugs!

Those who believe that anything "natural" must necessarily be healthier and better for us than anything manufactured in a laboratory will probably fall for these kinds of claims. And what could be more natural than something taken from the earth itself? According to some

MediScammers, virtually anything on the planet — if suitably marketed — could be used to cure what ails you. Following are some other examples.

CRYSTAL THEORIES ABOUND

Nothing typifies the gullibility of New Age medicine advocates more clearly than the belief in the presumed healing powers of crystals. Again, it starts with a modicum of science. In 1880 Pierre and Jacques Curie discovered that certain crystals, like quartz, produce an electric current when squeezed. This is called the "piezoelectric effect," and is what makes quartz watches and phonograph needles work. Thirty-five years later it was noticed that some crystals can be used to reflect or focus X rays and other wave forms. From this was derived the assumption that crystals can be used to focus mysterious "healing waves," or other presumed magical energy forms whose source and very existence cannot be demonstrated. Then again, why let science get in the way of a good theory? Just wearing a crystal, many believe, is all it takes to focus these healing waves in the right place—an idea akin to assuming that wearing a telescope lens around your neck would allow you to see the stars more clearly.

The BioElectric Shield

From such concepts evolved the BioElectric Shield, developed by a chiropractor who claims that the concepts behind his invention came from visions and voices in his head. The Shield—which is an arrangement of quartz crystals in a silver-and-brass amulet shaped like a flying saucer—is to be worn around the neck, and sells for $139 and up. According to company advertisements, "the Shield strengthens your energy field in two ways: first, by deflecting and redirecting energies that impinge on you from your environment, and secondly, by reinforcing your own natural energies so that they are much less susceptible to outside disturbances." Even if these claims were remotely true, you would have to encase your entire body in such crystals for them to offer such protection. The ad goes on to state that your strength is constantly sapped by exposure to electromagnetic radiation (which emanates from everything from battery-operated watches to TV remote controls), and that the BioElectric Shield is 99 percent effective in restoring this lost strength.

The Stimulator/Crystaldyne Pain Reliever

An even more outrageous use of crystals is the "Stimulator," also marketed as the "Crystaldyne Pain Reliever." Resembling a stubby hypodermic syringe, the product is supposed to eliminate pain without the use of drugs. According to advertisements, to make it work, "you apply Crystaldyne to the proper area, then push down on the red plunger. Inside, two special crystals impact to send a stimulus blocking signal to the pain site. You feel a slight, totally harmless tingle and the treatment is done!" The device could be used to relieve headaches, back pain, arthritis, stress, nosebleeds, and a host of other problems. Not only that, said the advertisements, but when "you use Crystaldyne with a partner, you can extend the stimulus effect by applying the device to one area then 'grounding' it by touching another area of your body. The stimulus effect will then pass from point to point." An interesting concept, although I have absolutely no idea what it is supposed to mean.

Neither, apparently, did the federal government. According to the *FDA Consumer*'s "Alert on the Stimulator," "The Stimulator is essentially an electric gas barbecue grill igniter outfitted with finger grips. When pressed against the skin, the device sparks and causes a small electric shock." The devices cost an estimated $2 to manufacture, yet were sold for a list price of $69.95. The FDA stepped in and stopped the company on the basis that they were marketing an unproved medical device. When 1,200 customers failed to receive the devices for which they had already paid, the company accused the FDA of having confiscated and cashed the checks that had been mailed in on those unfilled orders.

Herbal Crystallization

This unlikely test has been advertised as a discovery that takes the guesswork out of the prescribing process. It consists of adding a solution of copper chloride to a dried specimen of the patient's saliva, then examining the resulting crystal pattern under a microscope. This crystal pattern is then matched to the patterns of eight hundred dried herbs to decide which of the patient's bodily systems have problems and which herbs should be used to treat them.

If two parallel lines of crystals are noticed, they can be interpreted as representing a blood vessel. Garlic is usually recommended when this pattern appears, since garlic has "beneficial effects on the blood." According to registered dietitian Ellen Coleman, who wrote about this therapy for the "Healthcare Reality Check" Web site, there is absolutely no scientific basis whatever to this form of testing.

The Polarizer

Another outrageous use of crystals was described in a recent column by Fort Worth, Texas, physician and health fraud debunker Timothy Gorski. He writes in *The Tarrant County Physician* about a device called "The Polarizer," which purportedly uses crystals to purify food. The device is described as being composed of silicon dioxide crystals "with six-faced regular prisms with equal-sided pyramids on top"—in other words, common, everyday quartz. According to the manufacturer, these crystals have an "intrinsic data field, electro-magnetic field or aura" that is supposed to "deactivate the poisonous influence of pathogens like viruses, bacteria, spores, fungus, and eggs of intestinal worms, which can be found in most of our food."

The company offered no scientific evidence to back up these claims, but instead suggested that "the simplest and most convincing way to test the effects of The Polarizer is the human sense of taste."

This device is not only fraudulent but could be downright dangerous, since it would almost certainly lead some customers to eat spoiled or tainted food on the mistaken assumption that the device had purified it. The good news is that after checking the promoter's Web site we found no information about The Polarizer. All that remained was their Liechtenstein address.

The Weirdness Continues

Despite crackdowns on the more egregious marketers, false and unproved claims about the magic powers of crystals never cease. Today there's even an academy in Hawaii which offers beginning, intermediate, and advanced courses in "crystal healing." These courses, which cost $600 apiece exclusive of required textbooks written by the academy's founder, teach prospective healers techniques like the "Laying On of Stones," and how to select crystals of the appropriate tune—from among "high octave" and "low octave" crystals—for treating each particular medical condition. Apparently crystal healing is a divine calling; those who finish the advanced course as well as a special teacher's training course become Ministers of the Crystalline Ministry.

BATHS AND SPRINGS

Claims of the curative powers of baths and hot springs precede even the times of the Romans. And the number of mineral or hot springs with presumed curative powers is far too great to list here. And they do appear to have some limited therapeutic benefit. After all, who among us hasn't at one time or another been relaxed and soothed by taking a long, hot bath? This is one area where there is in fact a substantial scientific basis underlying the claims of the promoters. But as we shall see, you don't need to leave your own community to take advantage of those benefits.

In the early eighteenth century, physicians reported that prolonged immersion in hot-water springs was particularly useful in treating *Colica pictonium,* a disease that was then common but is now virtually unknown. The disease was characterized by severe abdominal colic (paroxysmal pain), followed by trembling and a loss of sensation and control of the limbs. We now know that *Colica pictonium* was, in fact, a form of chronic lead poisoning brought about by the then widespread use of lead in cookware and eating utensils.

In 1920 experiments showed that prolonged immersion of the whole body up to the neck in water increases the production of urine, a process called diuresis. More recent experiments have shown that this diuresis is caused by water pressure. Simply put, the weight of the water exerts pressure on the lower body, squeezing water from the tissues into the blood. The deeper the water surrounding your feet and legs, the more intense the effect, so standing up is best. Internal pressure sensors in the blood vessels detect the increased fluid, triggering the kidneys to remove this excess fluid from the blood in the form of urine. The fact that patients were encouraged to drink copious quantities of the spring water while bathing in it further encouraged the production of urine, which in turn increased the rate lead was removed from the systems of the *Colica pictonium* victims, causing them to recover quicker.

Although lead poisoning today is rare and usually treated by chelation therapy, deep-water bathing appears useful in treating such disorders as edema and high blood pressure—again, by forcing the body to excrete excess fluids through urination. But you don't need to travel to some exotic destination to achieve these benefits, especially since the water doesn't have to be at any particular temperature or mineral content to bestow these benefits. Any lake, stream, swimming pool, or hot tub appears to work just as well. All you have to do to achieve these benefits is sit or stand up to your neck in water two or three times a week for up to three hours at a stretch.

DO-IT-YOURSELF CHEMOTHERAPY

A few years ago, the Pacific yew tree, *Taxus brevifolia*, was in the news as the source of the drug paclitaxel (marketed under the brand name Taxol), which is now used to fight breast, ovarian, and certain other forms of cancer. The drug was found in the bark of the Pacific yew tree, and there was concern at the time that the need for the drug might lead to a decimation of the yew trees. Since then, a means of manufacturing Taxol has been found that doesn't require harming the trees.

Enter next a company that began selling capsules, tinctures, salves, and tea bags made from the needles of the Pacific yew. Originally the company claimed its potions could cure cancer, arthritis, gall bladder and prostate disease—to name only a few. It was a dream come true. Chemotherapy in your own home for less than $50 a month—and you wouldn't even lose your hair.

Today, their Web site lists the same products as before, but makes much more conservative claims about their uses. Now the company Web site states only the fact that the Pacific yew has been the subject of intense cancer research, and leaves it to the shopper to infer what most of the yew-based products are to be used for. Interestingly, although the needles of the yew contain no paclitaxel, they do contain the related compound docetaxel, which does indeed have anti-cancer properties.

This raises important questions. Are cancer patients forgoing legitimate, physician-supervised cancer therapy in order to self-medicate with herbal extracts of unknown and potentially nonexistent anti-cancer properties? Alternatively, are they self-medicating in addition to standard cancer therapies, ingesting compounds that might potentially interfere with, or interact with, other drugs? As long as the company doesn't make any specific claims about the medicinal uses of their products, they are under no obligation to answer any of these questions.

COLLOIDAL MINERALS

The story behind the discovery of colloidal minerals is about as romantic as a MediScam ever gets. In the early years of the twentieth century, it goes, a cattle rancher in central Utah by the name of Thomas Jefferson Clark developed some unknown but serious malady. Clark was told about a healing stream by a Paiute medicine man and elder known as Chief Soaring Eagle. Supposedly the Paiutes had known about and benefited from these waters for centuries. Clark drank from the waters and quickly recovered his health. Intrigued by the miracle, Clark traced the stream back to its source in organic-rich shales. He experimented for several years with these shales, and by 1931 he had developed his own brand of tonic rich in these "colloidal minerals." And thus the legend began. The only drawback to this wonderful tale of discovery is that modern-day Paiutes have never heard of a Chief Soaring Eagle nor of any ancestral waters with healing powers.

A "colloid" mineral is simply one whose particle size is small enough to keep it suspended in a liquid but large enough to stop or delay its passage through a semi permeable membrane—the kind of membrane that surrounds every cell in our bodies. Even in theory, let alone clinical investigation, there is no reason to believe that this form of mineral would be nutritionally superior to the forms present in foods or generic multipurpose vitamin/mineral supplements.

The story of how colloidal mineral extracts are made is almost as interesting as the story of how they are promoted. The shales that Thomas Clark brought to light were originally laid down about 90 million years ago during the Cretaceous period. At the time, Utah was a place of dense tropical rain forests and fetid swamps. The shales laid down during that period were made from the clay, mud, and organic material called humus. These shales are interlaced with bituminous coal.

To make colloidal minerals, the shales (and a certain amount of coal) are first surface-mined, then ground to a powder. The powder is placed in stainless-steel vats, then covered with water and allowed to sit for several days while the minerals in the powder leach into the water. The bitter extract is then filtered and bottled.

Of course, the concept of drinking water that has been steeped in crushed rock that is filled with the remnants of rotted vegetation, which has been strip-mined out of an old swamp bed doesn't sound very appetizing. So the promoters describe the swamp as *ancient virgin rain forest,* the leach water as *natural,* and the deposits of rotted vegetation as *pristine.* You get the idea.

Naturally the promoters dismiss entirely the possible health dangers of their products. Scientist and author James Pontolillo points out that colloidal minerals, as currently processed, carry a number of distinct health threats. Hydrocarbons associated with coal, petroleum, and other fossil fuels carry a number of well-known health risks, including cancer.

And not all minerals are good for us, colloidal or not. Arsenic, lead, mercury, and cadmium—all toxic—are four of the seventy-five-odd minerals listed as coming from the shale leachate. Despite these dangers, colloidal minerals still can be sold as long as they are classified as dietary supplements and no specific medical claims are made for them. Buyer beware!

AROMATHERAPY

The problem with addressing aromatherapy is that it means different things to different practitioners. The most benign practitioners assert nothing more than that certain smells can effect desirable changes in mood. No problem there. Who among us hasn't felt a wave of pleasure when smelling our favorite meal cooking on the stove? And what's the point of the perfume industry if not to arouse desire? No doubt about it—aromas can and do elicit responses. But enough to *cure diseases?* At the other end of the spectrum are practitioners who maintain that aromatherapy can actually cure everything from high blood pressure to head lice. Just how far can one carry the concept of aromatherapy before becoming a MediScammer?

Although the basic concepts of aromatherapy have been around for centuries, the term itself did not come into use until 1928 when French chemist René Maurice Gattefossé published the book *Aromathérapie.* After a lab explosion, Gattefossé had plunged his badly burned hand into a vat of lavender oil. After noticing how quickly his hand healed, he began the investigations that led to the development of modern aromatherapy, which was revived by a pair of French homeopaths in the 1960s.

Aromatherapy centers around the use of essential oils of plant extracts. Essential oils are aromatic, volatile, and flammable. Some proponents have characterized these oils as containing the "soul" or "spirit" of the plants, and that the smell and appearance of the plant together reveal its "secret" healing properties. For example, because the appearance of the violet suggests modesty, they would hold that smelling violet oil imparts calmness and modesty.

Aromatherapists have suggested virtually every conceivable application path for essential oils: from bathing in water to which the oils have been added, to drinking teas of it, to massage or using suitably scented cosmetics. And the claims can be remarkable. One Los Angeles aromatherapy company claims that inhaling their scents "balances the biological background," "revitalizes the cells," and produces a "strong energizing effect on the sympathetic nervous system." Not only that, but the company claims that one of their products "promotes elimination of toxins and helps tone and firm the body." Another appears to act as an air filter, given that it is described as "ideal to rid the atmosphere of smoke and heavy odors." In 1997, NCRHI (The National Council for Reliable Health Information) filed suit against the company on the basis that it was violating the California Business and Professions Code by making false and misleading claims about its products. Although the original suit was thrown out, the NCRHI has appealed.

Most of the claims made by aromatherapists, however, are essentially non-testable, revolving around vague New Age concepts like "spiritual centering" and "soothing or sharpening the senses." And people who go for this kind of nonsense will probably go for the scents, too.

MAGIC WATERS

There are a lot of good reasons for drinking bottled water. Your tap water may have an objectionable odor or taste. Drinking fluoridated bottled water is better for children's teeth than unfluoridated well water. Conversely, some well water contains so much fluoride that it causes tooth discoloration. Those who live in older homes with original metal plumbing still installed may find that their tap water has an unpleasant metallic taste. The problem is not that bottled water is a bad idea, but that Medi-Scammers promote it for all the wrong reasons. And sometimes, the bottled water they promote is far worse for the customer's health than tap water. Here are some of the *wrong* reasons frequently given for drinking bottled water.

"Fluoride is bad for you." Fluoridation of municipal water supplies began after World War II, when it was realized that fluoride could reduce the incidence of cavities in children's teeth by up to 70 percent. As with many things in life, however, too much of a good thing can be worse than not enough. Besides tooth discoloration, excessive fluoride can cause a bone disorder called skeletal fluorosis. Anti-fluoridation activists have seized on this rare condition as an excuse to promote the use of bottled water. But government research has consistently shown that fluoride levels used in community water supplies pose no health risk, and the American Dental Association maintains flatly that "the overwhelming weight of scientific evidence indicates that fluoridation of community water supplies is both safe and effective."

Recent studies have found an increase in child tooth decay for the first time in twenty years. And it appears that the culprit is the increasing use of unfluoridated bottled water by families who use it exclusively for drinking and cooking. In response, some bottled water companies are now offering fluoridated water as an option.

"Chlorine is bad for you." Chlorine is added to almost all municipal water supplies to prevent the growth of algae, bacteria like *E. coli,* and parasites like cryptosporidium. An example of what can happen when water isn't properly chlorinated was shown in Milwaukee in 1993, when over 400,000 people became ill after the water supply became infected with cryptosporidium.

While some may find the smell and taste of chlorine objectionable, no one has yet come up with a valid, substantiated danger associated with drinking chlorinated water. And the benefits of having it in the water far outweigh the risks.

"Bottled water is a good source of minerals." Carrying this argument to the absurd extreme is one Arizona company. According to the company, they've discovered the secret to living to age one hundred and beyond in perfect health.

As stated in their promotional literature, there are at least five areas on Earth where people maintain perfect health and live naturally to one hundred or more years. How? The local inhabitants claim that it is their special water. These locations are all remote areas ranging from Tibet to Peru. The company claims it took them seventeen years to discover what makes the waters from these regions so remarkable: the water "comes from ice blue glaciers," and the "cloudy colloidal water found in these areas is full of natural colloids and organic polyelectrolytes." Fortunately for you, you don't have to travel to any of those exotic locations to avail yourself of these mineral miracles. All you have to do is drink their water.

The simple—and inexpensive—reality is that water is just one of many dietary sources of minerals, and depending on its source, your tap water may have as many, if not more, minerals than bottled "mineral water."

Although bottled water is normally touted as "pure" and "natural," it's estimated that between 25 and 40 percent of all bottled water is nothing more than filtered tap water. Further, a four-year study by the Natural Resources Defense Council found that one-third of all bottled waters tested had levels of contaminants—including arsenic, bacteria, and organic chemicals—that exceeded acceptable limits.

A more recent twist is "superoxygenated water," which is simply water that has had oxygen bubbled through it. Manufacturers of these products claim they freshen your breath, increase energy, stamina, and enthusiasm, and provide relief from fatigue and hypoxia. All these claims are hogwash, given that the amount of additional oxygen supplied by such beverages would be dwarfed by the oxygen present in a single breath of air.

The bottom line is that MediScammers will literally go to the ends of the earth to part you from your money. Fortunately, almost everything of any value they have to offer you is readily available in a cheap, generic form that offers all of the benefits of their products at a fraction of the cost and often with fewer risks. Know what it is that you're really buying, and learn to shut out the marketing claptrap.

chapter 9

Plastic Surgery— The MediScammers' Newest Target

The Price of Vanity Can Be Crippling—or Worse

SARAH H. PILZNER (not her real name) of Cooper City, Florida, knew that her breast augmentation surgery was a mistake the minute Henry Castillo, her self-proclaimed plastic surgeon, cut into her. Due to faulty anesthesia, she was still conscious and very much in pain. She begged Castillo to stop. He continued anyway.

The surgery took place in Castillo's private offices in a medical center in North Miami. Sanitary conditions were, to say the least, questionable. Castillo's chauffeur wandered into the operating room in street clothes just to watch the surgery. Without even washing his hands, he picked up a surgical instrument and handed it to Castillo. He then used a tissue to wipe the tears from Sarah's eyes.

The day after her surgery, the woman's breasts were swollen, painful, and oozing black fluid. She wound up in emergency surgery, where another plastic surgeon removed the implants and cured her infection. Outraged, the second surgeon called the police. The police called state health officials, who advised them that Henry Castillo was not licensed to practice medicine in Florida. The police soon had Castillo in custody, but not before he had maimed at least three women.

Although Castillo, forty-one, claimed to have studied medicine in Mexico, officials found no reason to believe he had any medical training at all. He was already on probation for a previous conviction for practicing medicine without a license. But his abuses went even deeper than that. One of the ways that Castillo had attracted patients was by promising to bill the entire cost of the surgery to their medical insurance. While cosmetic procedures are not usually paid by insurance, Castillo would simply falsify the insurance claim by labeling the surgery as something that *was* covered by insurance—breast augmentations, for example, were sometimes labeled as "cyst removal."

Eventually Castillo was charged with defrauding insurance companies of $140,000. In August of 1999 Castillo pleaded no contest to charges of racketeering, insurance fraud, and grand theft. In a plea bargain he was sentenced to three years in prison and ordered to pay restitution of $55,000. It's a sad commentary that all of the charges he was convicted on involved defrauding insurance companies, and were not for seriously injuring patients by practicing medicine without a license.

Castillo was only one of at least a dozen fake plastic surgeons that Fred Schulte and Jenni Bergal, reporters for the *Sun-Sentinel,* discovered practicing in south Florida. And the resulting horror stories can sound like something out of a pulp-fiction novel.

Take the case of Alexander Baez of Miami, Florida. He was a forty-seven-year-old champion bodybuilder who decided that his pectoral muscles just weren't big enough. He'd heard about a plastic surgeon by the name of "Dr. Reinaldo" who specialized in surgically enlarging female breasts and male pectoral muscles. Baez decided that, because the operation would enhance his career, the few thousand dollars it cost would be money well spent. So he went to Reinaldo's offices in trendy South Beach for the surgery.

During the operation, Baez woke up three times in excruciating pain and with tears in his eyes as Reinaldo tried to force an oversized implant into his chest with an object that looked very much like a kitchen spatula. And when Baez finally came out of anesthesia for the last time, he was told that everything was okay. He was sent home immediately.

But everything *wasn't* okay. Instead of getting a pectoral-muscle enhancement, he now had breasts. And the female breast implants Reinaldo had inserted in his chest were leaking. Police would soon discover that Baez wasn't the only victim of Reinaldo's outrageously incompetent surgeries. Their investigations would also reveal that "Dr. Reinaldo," who had been performing cosmetic surgeries in his South Beach office for over a year, was not a plastic surgeon. In fact, he wasn't any kind of doctor at all! He was a con man by the name of Reinaldo Silvestre.

The procedure itself was simple. Silvestre charged between $3,000 and $4,000 for each surgery. He drugged the patient with ketamine, an anesthetic commonly used on animals, then cut open the chest and inserted the implants. If the surgery was botched, Silvestre assured the patient that he could repair the damage. And many of his patients did come back, some of them more than once. He was so confident of his skills as a surgeon that he even allowed some of his surgeries to be video-taped, including the one on Baez. Detective Juan Sanchez of the Miami Beach Police Department described the video to me as "the most gross thing I've ever seen."

Silvestre's ruse was discovered when one of his female patients went to police after having endured several failed attempts to repair damage that had left her breasts drastically different sizes. She brought along a videotape of Baez's surgery as evidence. Silvestre was charged with practicing medicine and administering narcotics without a license, and aggravated battery. A class action suit was also filed against him by some of his victims. Silvestre soon disappeared, and as of this writing the police are still searching for him. Authorities are worried that if Silvestre is delusional and really does think he is a good surgeon, he might set up shop elsewhere.

Spencer Aronfeld, the attorney who represents some of the bogus plastic surgeon's victims in Miami, told me, "Silvestre is a criminal of the first degree. He left mangled and deformed bodies and broken promises on Miami Beach. He caused my clients severe and painful physical and emotional injuries, and one day I pray that I will be able to cross-examine him in a court of law in front of a jury." According to Aronfeld, Miami surgeon John Cassel, M.D., F.A.C.S., fixed the injuries of Aronfeld's clients for free.

Given the fact that training to become a plastic surgeon involves four years of medical school, five years of a general surgery residency, and another five years of specialty surgery residency, the question becomes: How could Silvestre have faked such extensive credentials for as long as he did and continued operating on patients?

Part of the answer is that Silvestre shared traits that have always distinguished the successful quack: charm and self-confidence. His office bore all the trappings of a successful practice, and his likable demeanor and easy smile quickly won his patients' trust. And for some patients, his betrayal of them was what hurt most. So how could his victims have protected themselves? A quick call to the state medical board would have revealed that there was no "Dr. Reinaldo" licensed to practice medicine anywhere in Florida.

THE UNDERESTIMATED DANGERS OF COSMETIC SURGERY

Pilzner and Baez are by no means the only patients ever maimed by a con artist posing as a plastic surgeon. Why didn't the victims of these quacks think twice? Perhaps plastic surgery is becoming too commonplace. Maybe we Americans are beginning to think of difficult and dangerous surgeries as merely routine. As we'll see, the dangers of cosmetic surgery are very real, even at the hands of a competent surgeon.

Liposuction. Liposuction is the process by which fat is literally sucked out of thighs, bellies, and buttocks using a long vacuum tube. It's become the most popular cosmetic surgery in the U.S., with more than 200,000 procedures done every year on Americans who find the pain and expense of surgery easier to endure than dieting and exercise. The number of people electing to undergo this procedure has increased 216 percent since 1992.

Liposuction is a legitimate surgery, and the vast majority of patients who undergo it feel the benefits were worth the money. Still, the risks are significant. According to a recent *USA Today* article, plastic surgeons voluntarily reported a death rate of 1 patient in every 5,000 who underwent liposuction between 1994 and 1998. Most of these operations were conducted in the physician's private offices. By comparison, a patient's overall risk of dying while undergoing *any* surgery in a hospital during that same period was between 1 in 100,000 and 1 in 300,000—and that includes patients who underwent open-heart surgery, brain surgery, and other high-risk procedures. Further, the real risks of liposuction are probably much higher, given that the mortality statistics were only compiled for plastic surgeons—the most competent group of physicians to offer this procedure. As will be discussed later, far less qualified physicians also offer this service, and their fatality rates are surely higher than those of plastic surgeons. Dr. Erwin Moss, the executive director of the New Jersey State Society of Anesthesiologists, told me that, "the death rate associated with liposuction is totally unacceptable."

It's important to note here that death may occur even when surgeons are following accepted medical procedures. The surgery itself carries certain inherent risks—many of which are poorly understood—even when conducted under ideal circumstances. When liposuction is conducted under less-than-optimal conditions, the rate of complications and death increases accordingly.

Some liposuction deaths have resulted after patients developed massive infections that evolved into septicemia (blood poisoning) or had other major complications as a result of improper sterilization of the equipment. For example, two women in Houston died from uncontrollable infections after undergoing liposuction performed by a gynecologist, not a plastic surgeon. The equipment had not been sterilized properly, and the women's infections were not diagnosed until it was too late to save their lives.

Because there is no mandatory or central reporting system for cosmetic-surgery deaths and complications, determining just how widespread such problems are is difficult.

Breast Surgery. Breast augmentation is the second-most-common cosmetic surgery, according to the American Society of Plastic Surgeons. Whether it is augmentation, reduction, or a lift, breast surgery is a valid treatment from which millions have benefited. Yet all of these procedures carry certain risks even at the hands of a competent surgeon, and these risks are frequently underestimated. The risks include shifting or hardening of the implants, rupture of implants, and compromised blood flow to the living breast tissue. These complications can result in poor healing, wounds reopening, tissue death, scarring, and poor appearance.

Despite these known risks, over 2 million women have had breast implants. The FDA banned the silicone-gel breast implant after recipients came forward with inexplicable autoimmune diseases involving arthritic conditions, swollen joints, and other evidence of tissue rejection. Even without an actual perforation in the implant itself, the implants often leaked. It's believed that tiny amounts of silicone travel throughout the body, causing tissue reactions and inflammation of the lymph nodes as well as other problems of toxicity. Although there is no clear evidence that implants cause major diseases, silicone gel has been found to cause cancer in animals in laboratory tests, and the implants may interfere with mammography readings.

Even saline breast implants, which have largely replaced silicone implants, have never been declared completely safe by the FDA. Despite the risks, 130,000 women received saline implants in 1999 alone. A recent study found that up to 27 percent of women who received saline implants had them removed within three years, usually because of the development of painful scar tissue, infections, or because the implant broke and leaked. The FDA recently concluded that it's possible that a substantial number of patients will require additional surgery to remove or replace their implants due to complications.

Even in the hands of a conscientious and fully qualified plastic surgeon, breast surgery sometimes goes wrong. In the hands of a quack, it can become your worst nightmare. A few years ago I appeared on Sally Jessy Raphael's talk show with a woman who identified herself only as "Vicky."

Vicky had undergone reconstructive breast surgery following injuries she had suffered years earlier from an explosion. After the legitimate doctor who had inserted her original implants retired, she wound up in the hands of a quack who convinced her that her implants had turned "as hard as rocks" and were blocking her heart. If she didn't have them cut out immediately, he told her, she would die. The "doctor" insisted upon $700 up front immediately to do the surgery. He told her he would replace her old implants with new ones covered with a translucent foam. What Vicky got instead were implants (possibly even her old ones) covered with carpet foam. That's right—pieces of the padding they use under carpets. When she awoke from the anesthesia, her "doctor" was gone, and she has not seen him since. Her own problems, however, had just begun.

The carpet foam was so toxic to her system that Vicky was hospitalized for liver failure. Her weight dropped to forty-seven pounds. When the nurses turned her over, they had to pick up her skin and drape it over her. She developed gangrene in eight places, requiring amputation of large sections of flesh on her buttocks, legs, and head. At one point, her family was told she had only twenty minutes to live. Although she did— barely—survive the ordeal, Vicky needed another $14,000 worth of surgery to repair the damage. Even after the subsequent surgery, she was left horribly scarred and chronically ill.

Face-lifts, Hair Replacement, etc.

In 1988, a sixty-six-year-old semi-retired exterminator went to a surgical center in Hialeah, Florida, for a face-lift and wrinkle removal. The surgery was performed by Dr. José Jurado. After a two-hour surgery, the man was taken on a gurney to the recovery area to recuperate from the anesthesia.

That evening, the patient was found to be in distress: he was pale, sweating, and having trouble breathing. He went into respiratory arrest and died despite efforts to resuscitate him. It was determined that he died because the flow of oxygen to his brain had been accidentally cut off during anesthesia. A detective investigating the scene found the center's operating room to be dirty, with blood and pieces of skin scattered around. An investigator for the Dade County Medical Examiner's Office noted "filth" and "general squalor" in the operating room. Jurado voluntarily gave up his medical license in 1991 in response to a state investigation into the man's death.

Even when the doctor is competent and does the job well, things still can go wrong. In 1979, Henry X. Marine (not his real name), went to a plastic surgeon in Lima, Ohio (not the real location), for treatment of his male-pattern baldness. The surgeon offered a surgical procedure that consisted of injecting specially treated human hair directly into the scalp. This procedure is not to be confused with *hair transplantation,* in which the patient's own living hair follicles are moved from one part of the scalp to another. The surgeon carefully explained to the patient that the hair he was injecting would not grow and would break off or fall out within three years; therefore periodic reinjections of new hair would be needed.

The plastic surgeon also explained that he was one of the few doctors in the world who injected hair into the scalp in this manner, that the procedure was new and experimental, and that the doctor therefore could not guarantee the results. Marine agreed and the hair was injected.

Marine was initially delighted with the outcome of the surgery, and came back regularly for reinjection of replacement hair. In 1983, however, the FDA banned the procedure for new patients. As a continuing patient, Marine was allowed to receive replacement hair injections. However, realizing that the FDA was about to ban hair injection outright, his plastic surgeon discussed a "scalp reduction" procedure in which sections of the bald scalp would be surgically removed and the hair-growing portion of the scalp would then be pulled over the area and sutured in place.

The scalp reduction was performed but, because of complications caused by the injected hair, Marine's scalp was left permanently scarred. He sued his surgeon for malpractice, but the court found that the doctor had given the patient every reasonable warning that the results of the various surgeries could fall short of expectations.

I could list many more horror stories, but they all serve to make the same point: Cosmetic surgery is far more dangerous than most of us are led to believe. Certainly all those ads for plastic surgery on television and in magazines downplay the very real risks that patients take. Don't be lulled into a false sense of complacency with words that describe the procedure as "routine," "simple," or "painless." Be aware of the risks and ask yourself if the potential benefits are really worth it.

UNQUALIFIED DOCTORS ARE SCRAMBLING TO OFFER VANITY SURGERY

There are no laws preventing any licensed physician from performing any surgical or other medical procedure that he or she sees fit—whether the doctor is appropriately trained and competent to offer such services or not. Because of that, there are literally hundreds, perhaps even thousands, of doctors performing plastic surgery with no more training than having attended a weekend seminar on a particular procedure. In a scathing series of articles in southern Florida's *Sun-Sentinel*, Fred Schulte revealed just how extensive this problem is. His research found that there were only about four hundred doctors in the state of Florida who specialized in plastic or cosmetic surgery. Yet the Yellow Pages and Internet directories for the state that showed at least 920 Florida doctors offered such services in 1999. And it's not just medical doctors who reach outside their true speciality. Schulte found five dentists advertising that they perform hair transplants, and three of them do liposuction.

What about breast enlargements? Among those offering this surgery were two Florida eye doctors and an anesthesiologist. And varicose vein removal? A Colorado podiatrist (foot doctor) offered physicians a course on this technique costing $995. The headline of his recruiting brochure asked doctors, "Could your practice use $75,000 in cash next year?" After a two-day training seminar, the attendants could go back to their practices and offer the service to their patients.

As was pointed out by *Miami Herald* columnist Carl Hiaasen, any doctor with a medical degree and a scalpel can legally start hacking away on the general public. So a bored dermatologist or a burned-out radiologist can take a short training course, then hang out a new shingle and try a hand at nose jobs, face-lifts, and liposuction. And all of these procedures can present life-threatening complications even when carried out by fully trained plastic surgeons.

OFFICE SURGERY—Going Behind Closed Doors

Most cosmetic surgeries are performed in the doctors' private offices. On the one hand, this keeps costs down because even hospital outpatient surgical centers can be horrendously expensive. On the other hand, the reason hospitals are so expensive is that they have all the facilities and staff needed to take care of you if something goes wrong.

A big problem with office-based surgery is the management of anesthesia. In a hospital, you'll be attended by either a doctor or nurse who is specially trained to not only keep you out of pain but to monitor your condition constantly and react at the first sign of trouble. In office surgeries, anesthesia is often managed by untrained or undertrained personnel who lack the skills and training to react appropriately when things go wrong. And the anesthesia equipment in doctors' offices is often bought second-hand from a hospital that sold it because it was no longer up to safety standards. Some doctors manage anesthesia themselves—at the same time they're performing the surgery. That's like trying to drive a semi and a dragster at the same time. Anesthesia and surgery both require the undivided attention of fully trained professionals.

An even greater problem is that office surgery allows incompetent surgeons to hide their activities from the rest of the medical community.

Because surgical malpractice suits usually name the hospital as well as the surgeon as defendants, hospitals have a financial incentive to police the surgeons on their staff and root out those deemed incompetent or unethical. Likewise, good surgeons have an incentive to get rid of the bad ones because bad surgeons drive up the cost of malpractice insurance, and the horror stories generated by their botched surgeries scare many patients away. Bogus or incompetent surgeons, by confining their surgeries to their private offices, don't have to worry about anyone looking over their shoulders and criticizing their performance.

The fact is, many surgeries performed in private offices should actually be done in a hospital. This is especially true for patients who are at high risk of suffering complications during surgery. Take the case of one Hialeah, Florida, woman who, at four feet eleven inches and 305 pounds, was an insulin-dependent diabetic. Her obesity and generally poor state of health placed her at terrible risk for complications during anesthesia. A consulting doctor approved the liposuction procedure for the woman on condition that it be performed in a hospital. However, her doctor chose to carry out the four-hour operation in his own offices. The woman went into respiratory arrest during the surgery and died of anesthesia-related complications.

Dr. Ervin Moss of the New Jersey State Society of Anesthesiologists believes that "the high death rate among patients undergoing liposuction may in part be attributed to the fact that there are few rules for office based surgery. Although the state of California has some regulations, there's a maximum of $250,000 that can be awarded for any malpractice suit." He told me that recently a plastic surgeon performing a breast augmentation in a California office ran out of the surgery suite screaming for help when the patient went into cardiac arrest. Such scenes would never occur in a hospital setting.

KNOW YOUR COSMETIC SURGEON

Perhaps more than in any other area of medicine, in cosmetic surgery you get what you pay for. The main reason that many of the patients I've discussed in this chapter wound up at the mercy of a quack is that they shopped for the lowest price, not the best quality. And most of the patients I've discussed wound up paying far more than if they had gone to a reputable, fully competent surgeon in the first place. So be smart. If you're in the market for cosmetic surgery, shop for quality, not discounts.

For starters, don't be swayed by advertisements. You're not shopping for a car or a new refrigerator—your body and your health are being put at risk. Competent doctors rely on their professional reputation and referrals from other doctors and satisfied patients to fill their schedules. Ask yourself, if the doctor is so good, why does he or she have to advertise?

Ask your family doctor for one or two solid referrals. Then do some research. Call your state board of medical examiners and make sure that the doctor you're considering is licensed to practice medicine in your state. Also ask whether the doctor has been formally disciplined. If so, that should be a tip-off. Verify the doctor's certifications through the American Board of Medical Specialties (1-866-ASK-ABMS or online at www.certifieddoctor.org). A doctor certified by the American Board of Plastic Surgery (ABPS) has graduated from an accredited medical school and has completed at least five years of additional residency—usually three years of general surgery and two years of plastic surgery. He must practice plastic surgery for two years and pass a set of written and oral exams. The American Society of Plastic Surgeons (ASPS) represents 97 percent of all physicians certified by the ABPS. Call 1-800-635-0635 for the names of qualified professionals in your area. If a doctor is also a member of the American Society of Aesthetic Plastic Surgery (ASAPS), he or she has practiced plastic surgery for at least seven years and is affiliated with a major medical institution. You can phone 1-888-272-7711 for a list of ASAPS members in your area. Most competent cosmetic surgeons will be board-certified in either plastic surgery or dermatology. Be leery of doctors from other specialties—they may have acquired their "skills" through one of those weekend training seminars.

Even if your surgery is to take place in the doctor's offices, ask about which hospitals the doctor has staff privileges in. Membership on an accredited hospital staff generally means that the physician is recognized by his or her colleagues as competent. Beware of the doctor who isn't on the staff of any local hospital. Chances are there's a very good reason. The doctor may not be competent enough to get on the staff, or may have been booted off for incompetence or misconduct. Further, if something were to go wrong during your surgery, you'd want a doctor who could admit you directly to the hospital and stay with you. You certainly wouldn't want to have your care turned over to a complete stranger in the middle of a crisis.

Find out how many times the doctor has done this particular surgery, and how many of these procedures he or she does on a weekly basis. Generally, the more practiced the surgeon is, the more likely you'll get a satisfactory result. This is one area where you definitely don't want to be the guinea pig for a doctor who's just learning a new skill.

Next, call the hospital and ask if the doctor has privileges to perform the specific surgery you're considering. For example, if you're considering liposuction, you would want a surgeon who has liposuction privileges at that hospital, whether your procedure will be done in the hospital or not. You may find, for example, that your doctor has privileges for delivering babies and performing gynecological surgery, but not for doing liposuction. Why is this important? It's a gauge of the doctor's competence in that particular procedure. Occasionally a high-risk patient will need to be treated in the hospital instead of the doctor's office. A truly competent physician will be able to handle this situation because he or she has demonstrated before a panel of colleagues the needed skills and knowledge to perform such procedures even on high-risk patients. Those who are not fully trained and competent in a given procedure, on the other hand, probably wouldn't be allowed to perform it in the hospital.

Find out who the doctor's malpractice insurance carrier is, then call the carrier to verify that the doctor really is insured. Granted, you don't expect to use it. But it's like auto insurance, which you carry and expect the other drivers on the road to carry as well. If you're injured as the result of physician negligence, you want to make sure that there will be money available to compensate you and also to pay another physician to repair the damage. Be wary of the physician who doesn't carry malpractice insurance, just as you'd be suspicious of a driver who doesn't carry collision insurance. Too often, the reason they don't carry insurance is that they either can't afford it or can't get it in the first place because of a history of excessive claims against them.

Ask for patient testimonials. Meet face-to-face with at least one patient who's undergone the same procedure you're considering. Is the patient happy with the results? Would you be happy with the same outcome? And don't rely just on before-and-after photos. Photos won't tell you whether the patient was satisfied. They won't even tell you if the doctor you're considering was the one responsible for that particular surgery in the first place.

Finally, take a look around the office and operating facility. Does everything look clean and professional? A common theme repeated by many patients who suffered at the hands of quack plastic surgeons is, "I should have known something was wrong because everything was so dirty and shoddy."

Cosmetic surgery is a big investment. Certainly, it's a monetary investment. Except for reconstructive surgery, you'll almost always have to pay for it out of pocket. And you'll have to pay *a lot* of money—usually up front. That's the very factor that makes cosmetic surgery so attractive to MediScammers in the first place. More importantly, however, cosmetic surgery is a big investment of your hopes and dreams—and your health. So before you start forking over your money and entrusting your appearance and your health to any doctor, invest something else—the time and effort it takes to make sure that you'll be getting what you pay for.

chapter 10

Potent or Placebo?

Will the Real Cures Please Stand Up?

FEW THINGS IN MEDICINE are more intriguing than the concept of the placebo, which is Latin for "I shall please." Most of us think of a placebo as a sugar pill or sham injection intended to deceive the patient into thinking that he or she is getting real medication. In reality, the placebo is far more complicated and often includes therapeutic procedures that even legitimate physicians may falsely believe are medically beneficial. Placebos can involve almost any treatment method, ranging from simple psychological suggestion to fake surgery. And the results from a placebo can be stunningly effective. That is why, as we shall see, the placebo effect can pave an eight-lane highway connecting MediScammers to your wallet.

One researcher, on reviewing twenty-six medical studies that had used placebos, found that about one-third of all patients given a placebo will show some improvement, regardless of the illness. Sometimes the numbers can be much higher. The review of placebo studies by A. H. Roberts et al. in *Clinical Psychology Review* concluded that "under conditions of heightened expectations, the power of nonspecific effects (placebos) far exceeds that commonly reported in the literature." For example, initial research involving several treatments originally thought effective against herpes infections revealed that 85 percent of the patients in those studies reported "good" to "excellent" results, even though all of these treatments were later found to be useless.

Similar results can be found in surgical patients. One study found that about one-third of patients undergoing exploratory surgery to discover the source of lower-back and leg pain reported complete relief of their pain—even though the type of surgery they received provided no therapeutic benefit. Another study found that many patients suffering from angina pectoris (chest pain due to inadequate oxygen supply to the heart) showed substantial improvement after receiving a sham surgery that consisted of nothing more than making an incision in the skin.

Patient compliance has an important influence on the placebo effect, just as it does with real medications. In other words, patients who follow their doctor's instructions—even when those instructions are to take a placebo—do better than patients who don't follow such instructions. In one study in which patients with heart disease were given a placebo, the patients who took less than 80 percent of their placebo capsules had a 60 percent higher death rate over the next five years than the patients who took more than 80 percent of the placebo capsules.

Placebo effects also can be negative. While patient and physician confidence in a treatment can enhance its effectiveness, a lack of confidence can have the opposite effect. Patients have reported every manner of side effect in response to a placebo (these reactions are also referred to as the "nocebo" effect). Some patients actually develop hives, itching, edema, and other symptoms of allergic reaction in response to taking substances to which they are not otherwise allergic.

More importantly—and something that is not widely recognized—is that placebos actually can be harmful. The placebo response may convince a well patient that he actually has the disease for which he is being "treated" (see "Phony Diagnoses" later in this chapter). This situation can be used to convince patients that their imaginary disease is only amenable to the specific treatment offered by a MediScammer.

In legitimate clinical situations, true placebo use is usually restricted to research settings. Still, most physicians use placebos in some form, often unknowingly. Take, for example, the widespread practice of giving vitamin B12 shots to patients complaining of everything from fatigue to arthritis. Physicians know full well that very few patients actually suffer from B12 deficiency. They also know that the B12 shot will do no harm, and that many of their patients report feeling better and having more energy after getting one. Another consideration is that many patients feel cheated if the doctor gives them nothing more than advice; a B12 shot provides the patient something to "show" for the time and money spent going to the doctor.

HOW PLACEBOS WORK

An important component of the placebo effect is the power of suggestion, which usually leads to the patient's anticipation of a good result. Generally, the stronger this expectation, the more likely the patient is to report improvement. The strength of the expectation, in turn, depends on the personality of the patient. Those with dependent personality traits, who readily believe the doctor is fully in charge of the situation and is going to cure them, are more likely to react favorably to a placebo than those with more independent and suspicious personalities. The strength of the physician-patient relationship also plays a role here. If the patient likes and trusts the doctor, and if the doctor projects confidence in the cure, the patient is more likely to respond positively to almost any treatment, real or placebo. Some patients may actually improve just in order to live up to the doctor's expectations. Patients can even become addicted to placebos and may feel great distress if denied their "medicine."

The simple process of undergoing treatment also affects patient expectations. Psychiatrists have often compared their own profession to that of witch doctors, in that the healing processes of both are markedly similar. For both professions, the healing begins when the patient simply recognizes that a problem exists and seeks help. The next important step is when the healer puts a name to the problem—be it bipolar disorder or the evil eye. The simple naming of the problem gives the patient a measurable feeling of relief: Now that the healer has figured out what is causing the symptoms, he or she surely knows how to alleviate them. At that point, virtually any treatment—be it a prescription drug or rubbing the patient with a hen's egg—will result in substantial improvement. How? The most likely explanation is that the treatment process causes the body to release endorphins—naturally produced chemicals similar to morphine—that promote a sense of well-being. And the patient who feels better naturally thinks that he is being cured.

A second component of the placebo effect is spontaneous change. Many ailments are self-limiting. Most infectious diseases run their course over a few days. Chronic diseases, like arthritis, allergies, and gastrointestinal problems are cyclical, resulting in a roller-coaster ride of periodic degeneration and recuperation. If the patient takes a placebo about the time he begins to get better on his own, the placebo gets the credit. And because most patients seek medical help about the time their symptoms have peaked and spontaneous healing or remission is about to begin anyway, it's really not so surprising that the placebo effect is as strong and as common as it is.

Of course, the converse is also true: If the patient spontaneously develops a stomachache or has trouble sleeping, the placebo is blamed for the unwanted "side effects." However, since most patients are going to get better anyway around the time they take a placebo, their most likely reaction to the placebo is positive; MediScammers also understand this fact, and they know all too well how to take advantage of it.

QUACKERY AND THE PLACEBO EFFECT

Whether they honestly believe they are helping their patients or are purely in it for a quick buck, one trait above all else distinguishes MediScammers: They are good salespeople. In pitching their phony therapies, they not only lend credence to their own bogus theories, but they cast aspersion on the treatments offered by legitimate medical science.

Herein lies the crucial difference between quackery and scientific medicine. Science, by its very nature, is reserved and conservative. If you read the medical literature about a new drug being developed, you will rarely—if ever—see comments like, "Drug X cures disease Y." Instead, you will see careful, cautious comments such as "Drug X *appears effective* in treating disease Y," or "Drug X *may be clinically beneficial* in the treatment of disease Y." Why do scientists do this? *Because they know they may be wrong!* And they don't pretend otherwise. Therefore, the legitimate medical scientist will be the first to point out the possible errors and flaws in the research being reported. Only after years of careful research will the scientist commit to comments like, "Drug X has been shown to be clinically effective against disease Y."

The problem here is that, because scientists are themselves circumspect and constantly questioning their own results, they don't inspire the kind of patient confidence that contributes to the placebo effect. Nor, for that matter, would they even want to. Ask legitimate researchers whether their proposed treatment will help you, and the most likely answer will be, "I don't know, but I think it might." The medical scientists of the world want legitimate therapies that work, regardless of the patient's attitude. At least during the investigational phase of drug development, the placebo effect is not the scientist's friend, but the enemy—because it obscures what may or may not be the treatment's true effect on the patient.

Enter now the quacks, the MediScammers. Because all they have to sell are placebos, without the placebo effect their "cures" quickly would be revealed as fraudulent; therefore the quacks must play the placebo effect for maximum possible impact. This means they must be super salespeople capable of making patients believe in even the most outlandish claims. They point out the limitations of legitimate medicine, exploiting the caution and self-criticism of medical scientists to the quack's own benefit, claiming that they have the "real" cure. They promise whatever the audience wants to hear, offering hope to the incurable and relief to those in pain. The patient is told, without doubt, that what the MediScammer offers is exactly what the patient needs. So the patient puts up the money and, sure enough, reports feeling better almost immediately. And the MediScammer has yet another testimonial to add to his sales pitch—all thanks to the placebo effect.

Following is only a partial listing of some recent or ongoing MediScams that rely on the placebo effect to part the gullible from their money.

PSYCHIC SURGERY AND SPIRITUALISM

Nothing illustrates the placebo effect—and human gullibility—better than the "psychic surgeons" of Brazil and the Philippines. These quacks, who have no medical training and often little more than an elementary education, claim to be able to perform surgery with their bare hands without the use of anesthetics or antiseptics, and leave behind absolutely no scar or other sign that the skin was entered.

In reality, the "surgery" is a sleight-of-hand in which the supposed surgeon palms a capsule of red liquid resembling blood which he breaks open as he "enters" the skin. The blood immediately starts dripping from the "incision," giving the appearance the surgery is real while at the same time obscuring from onlookers what is really going on. Pressing his fingers hard against the soft tissue of the abdomen (and keeping spectators and their cameras at a distance), the psychic surgeon next makes it appear as if he is exploring the patient's internal organs with his bare hands. Then he produces a piece of flesh or some other item—also palmed— as the "tumor" that has now been safely removed. The blood is then washed off and the patient is magically restored.

Although this MediScam is strictly prohibited in North America (which is not to say that it doesn't happen), tour agencies often organize groups of desperate patients from Europe, Japan, the U.S., Australia, and New Zealand to visit the psychic surgeons on their own turf. Usually these patients are so anxious for treatment that they're willing to try anything, no matter how far-fetched. The late comic Andy Kaufman was one of the more famous victims of these MediScammers. He'd sought treatment for his inoperable lung cancer in the Philippines, and died from the disease a few weeks after being "operated on" by psychic surgeons.

Psychic surgeons claim to be able to treat a wide variety of ailments ranging from diabetes to cancer. And many patients do in fact report miraculous improvement, especially for poorly defined, nonspecific disorders like headaches, abdominal pain, and backaches. As for the psychic surgeons, they make no bones about their use of the placebo effect. They openly claim that the primary benefit of their surgery is to restore the patient's faith and confidence in the natural healing process, and therefore what the psychic surgeons do is morally no different from a Western doctor giving a placebo. In a magazine interview, Reverend Tony Agpaoa, one of the most famous of the psychic surgeons, stated flatly that his patients heal themselves. Said Agpaoa, "I merely plant the seed with my surgery. The patient's mind does the rest."

Perhaps a good thing to keep in mind is something that Ben Franklin wrote in *Poor Richard's Almanac* in 1736: "God heals, and the doctor takes the fees."

Psychic surgery is only one of many MediScams that have developed a cult following through a combination of religion, mysticism, and bogus medical knowledge. Unlike psychic surgery, however, most of these cults center around only one or two individual "healers."

Take the case of "Dr. David" who, in the mid-1990s, broadcast over a Medford, Oregon, radio station a weekly Spanish-language program aimed at an audience of mostly migrant farm workers from Mexico and Central America.

Dr. David, actually a twenty-four-year-old native of Colombia by the name of Geovanny Gutierrez-Montoya, knew exactly how to prey on the hopes and fears of his listeners, whose deep-rooted beliefs combined traditional Catholicism with Native American spiritualism and demonology. His radio messages were ominous and forbidding to a people who didn't need any more bad luck in their lives.

"There are people out there who are looking to hurt you," Gutierrez-Montoya told his audience. "They are looking to cause you catastrophe, destruction."

It sounded horrible—worse, it sounded true. These were a people brought up to believe that black cats and buzzards were to be feared, and that the world was alive with dark forces. But unlike gringo physicians who laughed at such things, Dr. Davíd was a *curandero,* a healer. More importantly, he was one of them. He understood the reality of their fears.

"It's dangerous," Gutierrez-Montoya assured them, "but we will protect you from bad energy. So I suggest that you come to my astrological center, the Family of Faith."

Gutierrez-Montoya's "Family of Faith" center was located in a small, second-floor office in Medford. Visitors—and he had more than twenty between January and April 1995—were charged $40 for a half-hour initial consultation. During that consultation they were usually told that their problems were far worse—much darker and more mysterious—than they ever could have guessed. When one migrant worker stepped in complaining of a sore back, for example, he was warned that his teenage son was destined to be paralyzed in a car wreck. The only way to prevent this was for him to buy and burn nine candles made in Rome out of human body fat.

The migrant asked how much the candles would cost.

"A hundred and fifty dollars a candle," Gutierrez-Montoya told him.

In all, the most impoverished of Medford's citizens paid more than $20,000 over a four-month period for Gutierrez-Montoya's mystical advice, incense, and candles. And it wasn't just money being wasted. One woman, a diabetic, died shortly after Gutierrez-Montoya advised her not to see a physician. Although some of his followers were beginning to question what they saw, Gutierrez-Montoya advised them that they would go blind and become mute if they went to the cops.

It was all, of course, a scam. Dr. Davíd was neither a holy man nor physician. But since he wasn't exactly practicing medicine in the Western sense of the term, it would be difficult for prosecutors to prove that he was treating patients without a license. In fact, the district attorney maintained, it would be difficult to prove his actions weren't protected under the constitutional guarantees of freedom of religious expression.

On the other hand, Gutierrez-Montoya *was* prescribing and selling candles he claimed were made of human fat. If they weren't, it would be fraud, pure and simple. That's the point where my production team and I linked forces with the Medford Police Department and the Immigration and Naturalization Services (INS) to bust Gutierrez-Montoya as a Medi-Scammer.

Our bait was Maria Swann, a meek-acting woman who went to Gutierrez-Montoya with the story that she had had her fallopian tubes tied, but now desired to have a son. Sitting in Gutierrez-Montoya's dimly lit office, Maria was assured that she could have a son. But first she would have to buy four of his human-fat candles—at $900 apiece. Maria asked to see the candles. The thin young man with a wispy mustache leaned forward over his desk.

"I cannot show you the candles because I've already lit them," Gutierrez-Montoya told her. "And nobody goes in where they are. Nobody, not even the wind enters. It's a dark place, very dirty; it smells horrible, eternally horrible."

Gutierrez-Montoya gave her a series of instructions that included having sex with her husband with someone watching, then bringing a condom filled with her husband's semen for Gutierrez-Montoya to "treat" before placing in her vagina.

A week later, Maria returned with a condom supposedly bearing her husband's semen (actually, it was white liquid dish soap). Gutierrez-Montoya told her that spirits would take control of her body, and that the body she would feel against hers would actually be her husband's. Gutierrez-Montoya then told her to undress. That's when the police and INS officers barged in, followed by me and my camera crew.

Ultimately Gutierrez-Montoya was charged with a Class C felony and served only two months in jail. He was then released on the condition that he devote six months to help the police nail other con artists similarly scamming the Hispanic community.

HOMEOPATHY

While not all homeopathic treatments rely on the placebo effect, most of the "medicines" used by its practitioners certainly do.

Homeopathy was founded in the early nineteenth century by the German physician Samuel Hahnemann, who was rightly concerned that many of the drugs and procedures employed by physicians of the day did more harm than good. Hahnemann declared that diseases represented a disturbance in the body's ability to heal itself. He went on to describe the source of disease as a suppressed itch, called the "psora." From this he developed the "law of similars," which holds that healing can be stimulated in the patient by administering infinitesimally small amounts of substances that, when administered in large doses to healthy people, produce symptoms similar to those of the disease. For example, if the patient suffers from nausea, you would treat him with minute amounts of a substance that can make healthy people nauseous. Hence the name "homeopathy," from the Greek words for "similar" and "disease."

Homeopathic "remedies" are made from herbs, minerals, and other substances that are mixed with water or alcohol, then diluted to fantastic extremes, equivalent to less than one drop of the original substance in an Olympic-sized swimming pool. Unlike scientific medicine, in which stronger drug doses are usually found to be more clinically effective than weaker doses, homeopathy holds that the more dilute the medicine, the better it works. The dilution involves a vigorous mixing process called "succussing," plus "potentizing" by tapping the mixing container with the heel of the hand or a leather pad. The concept is that the water molecules are supposed to retain a "memory" of the original substance, and through this stimulate the immune system.

Although homeopathic physicians claim that their healing methods are supported by an abundance of studies and published research, virtually no legitimate scientist recognizes these studies as valid—largely because of their failure to factor out the placebo effect. Properly controlled studies conducted by the mainstream medical and scientific communities have invariably found homeopathic medicines to be totally useless.

LAETRILE

Laetrile is chemically related to amygdalin, a substance originally isolated in France in 1830. In the presence of certain enzymes, amygdalin releases poisonous hydrogen cyanide. German physicians tried using this substance as a cancer treatment as early as 1892, but discarded it as ineffective and too toxic.

In the 1950s Ernst T. Krebs Sr., M.D., and his son Ernst Jr., a medical-school dropout who nonetheless used the title "Doctor," began using a form of "purified" amygdalin they named "Laetrile" to treat patients with cancer. They claimed that cancer cells are rich in an enzyme that causes Laetrile to release cyanide, which in turn destroys the cancer cells. Healthy cells, they said, are protected from injury by a different enzyme that deactivates the cyanide. There is no scientific basis to either of these claims.

By the late 1950s the mainstream medical community was beginning to take notice of Laetrile, both because of publicity generated by the Krebs and because of patient testimonials. However, when the Cancer Commission of the California Medical Association reviewed the charts of patients treated with Laetrile, they could find no evidence anyone was being helped by the drug. Likewise, animal tests at three medical centers using Laetrile found the drug to be totally ineffective.

In its official report, issued in 1963, the Cancer Advisory Council of the California Department of Public Heath stated that Laetrile was "of no value in the diagnosis, treatment, alleviation, or cure of cancer." Very shortly thereafter, and in spite of vigorous protests of Laetrile supporters, the drug was banned from use in the state.

With the FDA preparing to crack down on Laetrile nationwide, Krebs Jr. now began claiming that it was actually a vitamin—B17—and that cancer was caused by a deficiency of B17. The ploy failed. Laetrile's proponents simply packed up and moved across the border to Tijuana, Mexico, where cancer clinics continue to offer the treatment to this day. But Laetrile seekers need look no further than their computers. Laetrile drug products are readily available on the Internet as amygdalin or vitamin B17.

The main problem with most quack remedies is that they convince the patient to forgo legitimate treatment, wasting the patient's time and money. Certainly Laetrile does this. But even worse, because it releases cyanide into the system, it actually interferes with other cancer treatments. And saddest of all, autopsies of some patients who have taken Laetrile reveal that cyanide poisoning contributed to their deaths.

In an interesting side note to the Laetrile story, Ernesto Contreras, M.D., a former pathologist who began offering Laetrile therapy in his Tijuana clinic in 1959, acknowledged in 1974 that few of his cancer patients were "controlled" with Laetrile, according to an article by Benjamin Wilson, M.D. He further acknowledged that only about 30 percent showed a "definite" response to the drug—exactly what could be expected from the placebo effect alone.

THERAPEUTIC TOUCH

Therapeutic Touch (TT), still widely used in nursing practice, was conceived in the early 1970s by Dolores Krieger, Ph.D., R.N., a faculty member at New York University's Division of Nursing. Although the practice is rooted in mysticism, its practitioners insist that it has a scientific basis. They claim the ability to heal or improve many medical conditions by using their hands to manipulate a "human energy field" perceptible above the patient's skin. According to TT theorists, this field resembles a "magnetic fluid" or "animal magnetism"—something first postulated by eighteenth-century charlatans. Practitioners also insist that they can detect illnesses and stimulate recuperation through their intention to heal. And they claim to do this without having to actually touch the patient.

The claims of TT's proponents are legion, with many testimonials to its healing powers. It has gained widespread acceptance by the nursing community, and the North American Nursing Diagnosis Association recognized it as the only treatment for the "energy-field disturbance" diagnosis. Other scientific nursing journals and societies came to recognize TT, and the American Nurses Association even held TT workshops at its national conventions. Proponents of TT claim that more than 100,000 people worldwide have been trained in the technique, including at least 43,000 health care professionals.

All these claims came crashing to earth after nine-year-old Emily Rosa of Colorado put TT to the test for a science fair project. In her experiment, twenty-one TT therapists stuck their hands, palms up, through a screen where they could not see what Emily was doing. In a randomized trial—decided by the flip of a coin—Emily held one of her own hands over one of the therapist's, then asked which of the therapist's hands was closest to Emily's. If TT practitioners were actually able to detect an energy field as claimed, they should have been right 100 percent of the time. By pure chance alone, they should have scored 50 percent. In reality, they were right only 44 percent of the time. Emily's results were published in the April 1, 1998, edition of *JAMA*. And, true to form of MediScammers everywhere, the founders of TT cried foul and argued that Emily's experiment was biased and unfair. To be fair, most practitioners of TT appear to honestly believe they are offering a legitimate therapeutic service. However, by definition, scientific medicine demands that any acceptable therapy be reproducible by independent practitioners, whether they believe in the therapy or not. If we consider results that cannot be independently reproduced to be a Medi-Scam, then TT is a MediScam.

PHONY DIAGNOSES

Even when their MediScam can't cure any known disease, true quacks won't stop there. They'll invent their own disease! After all, everybody has some symptoms of some kind—occasional sleeplessness, headaches, morning stiffness, whatever. All you have to do is loop together a handful of symptoms—preferably vague ones common to the normal aging process so a lot of people will be affected by them—then assign a new name to the "syndrome." And because the MediScammer is the only one to recognize the existence of this syndrome—guess what?—he's the only one with a cure for it!

Stephen Barrett, M.D., who maintains the Web site known as "Quackwatch" (www.quackwatch.com), calls these "fad diagnoses." Whereas medically recognized diagnoses are associated with a clear-cut history, physical findings, and laboratory tests, says Barrett, fad diagnoses are associated with an endless variety of vague symptoms and typically do not correlate with any physical findings or scientific laboratory tests. The treatment of such disorders almost always involves vitamin and mineral supplementation. Some recent fad diagnoses he lists include:

- **Candidiasis hypersensitivity or yeast allergy.** According to proponents, 30 percent of Americans suffer from this "problem," said to be caused by a weakening of the immune system from yeast-derived products ranging from antibiotics to bread. Treatment involves the removal of such products from the diet, antifungal drugs, and vitamin and mineral supplementation.

- **Cavitational osteopathosis.** Some dentists maintain that everything from heart disease to arthritis is caused by infected "cavitations" within the jawbone that cannot be detected by X rays or treated with antibiotics. They advocate locating and scraping out the infected tissues and sometimes removing teeth from the area. As we'll see in chapter 13, there is no scientific evidence to support either the diagnosis or treatment of such a condition.

- **Electrical hypersensitivity.** The cause of this presumed disorder is exposure to electromagnetic fields, ranging from TV sets to overhead power lines. Symptoms attributed to such exposure include fatigue, weakness, nonspecific aches and pains, and irregular heartbeat. Treatment varies, but includes homeopathy, chiropractic, acupuncture, vitamin and mineral supplementation, and avoiding electrical fields.

- **Leaky Gut Syndrome.** According to proponents, this is caused when the lining of the gut is disturbed, allowing "unwanted substances" to penetrate the gut and enter the bloodstream. The body responds by producing antibodies, and this can result in everything from arthritis to chronic fatigue syndrome to lupus. Treatment includes avoiding processed foods, and vitamin and mineral supplementation.
- **Mercury-amalgam toxicity.** This is the belief that mercury-amalgam ("silver") fillings are toxic and cause a wide range of health problems ranging from Parkinson's disease to arthritis. Research has found that the mercury absorbed from dental fillings is insignificant. This is another topic we'll be taking a closer look at in chapter 13.
- **Multiple chemical sensitivity (MCS).** Basically, this theory holds that exposure to environmental chemicals, ranging from auto exhaust to perfume, produces multiple symptoms that include sleep and concentration disorders, chronic fatigue, memory loss, migraines, and allergy symptoms. Treatment involves minimizing exposure to chemicals, and vitamin and mineral supplementation.
- **Sick building syndrome.** Usually linked with MCS, this one holds that toxic fumes build up in our homes and offices due to insufficient ventilation. Treatment is the same as for MCS.

Barrett goes on to list the formula for creating your own fad disease, which includes making claims that millions of people suffer from it but are undiagnosed, picking a few treatments that allow unscrupulous chiropractors and health food stores to cash in on the action, promoting your ideas in books and on talk shows, and claiming that the medical establishment and drug companies are conspiring to suppress your research. Finally, if your claims are challenged, say that you're too busy taking care of sick people to mess with research, and that your clinical results speak for themselves.

How does all this tie into the placebo effect? Let's refer back to the earlier discussion in this chapter about what many claim are similarities between psychiatrists and witch doctors. Remember that the patient's placebo effect begins with the simple act of seeking care, and solidifies when the practitioner puts a name on the problem. All of a sudden, thanks to the phony diagnosis, those aches and pains that have been plaguing the patient for years have a *name;* and because the symptoms and findings associated with the diagnosis are deliberately vague, it's nearly impossible to prove that the patient *doesn't* have the named syndrome. As for the cure or treatment to this mystical disease—you can bet the farm that the MediScammer has one, and that it doesn't come easy or cheap.

COLONIC DETOXIFICATION

Although the methods of colonic detoxification take several forms, the rationale behind most of them involves the theory of "autointoxication." According to this theory, stagnation of bodily wastes in the colon (large intestine) causes toxins to form. These toxins are then absorbed and poison the body. Some proponents go so far as to say that hardened feces may accumulate on the colon wall for months or even years, compounding the problem by blocking food absorption and causing wastes from the blood to be reabsorbed by the body. Every one of these assumptions was proven baseless decades ago.

The reality is that most nutrient absorption takes place in the small intestine, that the colon acts mainly to transport wastes to the rectum for elimination and to absorb minerals and water, and that there is no evidence whatever that hardened feces accumulate on the colon walls. Nonetheless, colonic-detoxification enthusiasts claim that death begins in the colon, and that 90 percent of all diseases are caused by improperly working bowels.

To rid the body of these supposed toxins, adherents of the autointoxication theory recommend fasting, "cleansing" the colon with various herbal compounds that usually include laxatives, and colonic irrigation.

The last is the most dangerous. This involves inserting a rubber tube twenty to thirty inches inside the colon, then pumping warm water in and out. More than twenty gallons of water may be used in these treatments, compared with about a quart used in normal enemas. Sometimes coffee, herbs, plant extracts, or other concoctions are added to the enema water. As with all MediScammers, the practitioners of this therapy can present testimonial after testimonial from repeat customers who swear—in all honesty—they have never felt better or had more energy since undergoing this treatment.

The danger is that the bowel can be perforated during the process. At least six patients have died from such injuries while undergoing colonic irrigation. Another danger is the transfer of disease-causing organisms from one patient to the next if the equipment is not properly sterilized. In one case, thirty-six people were infected with parasitic amoebas following irrigation by unsterile equipment.

Nor is the use of herbal laxatives or "colon cleansers" always safe. Stimulants like castor oil and cascara sagrada can damage the nerves lining the wall of the colon. This can decrease the normal contractions of the colon, reducing its ability to eliminate waste. And that, in turn, may increase the problems of chronic constipation. Those who abuse laxatives may well find themselves unable to have a bowel movement without them.

Yet, as with the other "remedies" described in this chapter, the placebo effect keeps patients coming back. In part, that's because many patients are unduly anxious about "irregularity," having been falsely convinced by MediScammers and television laxative ads that it is abnormal and unhealthy not to have a bowel movement every day. The truth is, many people have bowel movements only two or three times a week, sometimes less, with no ill effects. But for the adherents of colonic detoxification, the false sense of security that comes from regular bowel movements and a supposedly clean colon outweigh the very real dangers of the therapies they are indulging in.

THE HEALTHY SKEPTIC

Understanding the placebo effect is important for avoiding MediScams because it explains why bogus cures sometimes appear to work. It also explains why legions of honest patients will provide testimonials as to the effectiveness of even the most worthless treatment. A healthy skepticism toward patient testimonials about dubious-sounding "cures" is a good buffer to keep between your wallet and a MediScammer.

chapter 11

Nursing Homes . . . or Warehouses for the Elderly?

Surely Our Parents Deserve Better than This

EIGHTEEN-YEAR-OLD JUSTIN MARTIN beat an elderly defenseless woman in her bed and sexually assaulted her. Martin had not broken into her home, nor had he abducted her. Martin was an employee of a nursing home in Oklahoma where the woman lived. And she had been entrusted to his care. A helpless old woman had been delivered into the hands of a vicious sadist.

At first her family was perplexed. "She was bruised from head to toe," said her granddaughter. "And we just didn't know what had happened and what went wrong."

The family finally learned the truth after Martin burned the woman under his care with a cigarette lighter. Not just once, but again and again. But the family's awareness came too late. Two weeks after the burnings, she died.

In the end, the woman's family would successfully sue the nursing home for not investigating Martin's background. A key allegation of their case would be that the nursing home never should have hired Justin Martin in the first place. Martin hadn't tried to hide his dark past. When he applied at the nursing home, he listed a drug-rehabilitation center as his home address. Oklahoma law states that no nursing home can employ "a drug addict or convicted felon." The nursing home had not investigated Martin's background, even though by law they were supposed to clear all job applicants with the Oklahoma State Bureau of Investigation (OSBI) within seventy-two hours of hiring them.

SHODDY HIRING PRACTICES

The sad fact is the Justin Martin case is not uncommon. Across the country, helpless, bedridden nursing-home residents are being bullied, abused, and manhandled. Who are their so-called "caregivers," and how are they getting jobs in nursing homes?

I decided to find out just how easy it is to get a job in a nursing home. In January 1999 I went undercover for a national television show to find out how carefully nursing homes screen their employees.

I "borrowed" the identity of a real-life career criminal and ex-convict who had been in prison three times. His tally of crimes was as long as a grocery receipt. He had been convicted of everything from assault and burglary to receiving stolen property and grand theft.

Using the ex-convict's identity, I applied for jobs at several Oklahoma nursing homes. At my first stop, I had no chance; the facility checked with the OSBI. They were sorry, they told me, but they could not use me.

At the second nursing home, I met with a nice lady named Helen (not her real name). I filled out an application, and Helen hired me on the spot. Only then did she have me fill out the background check forms. Four days later I was on the job. I contacted the OSBI. They told me the second home had never submitted the proper forms, including the all-important Criminal History Information Request.

Next stop was a third nursing home, where I met with the owner. She told me of their strong reputation. "Part of that is because I have been so picky with my staff," she assured me. Still, she admitted that turnover was high. She needed people, so she hired me. And she, too, failed to check me out with the OSBI.

I was also hired at a fourth nursing home. I could start Monday, said the woman who hired me. She seemed overworked and flustered.

"What about all the forms I need to fill out?" I asked.

"All this stuff is stuff the federal government likes," she said, waving an arm as if to make all those nasty forms go away. "We spend half our lives pleasing them."

The fourth nursing home also failed to contact the OSBI.

My investigation led to the depressing conclusion that three out of these four nursing homes eagerly would have hired a potentially violent ex-convict. Hundreds of residents could have been in grave danger. What's more, the positions scarcely paid better than minimum wage. A thief might be tempted to "supplement" this income at the expense of the residents by stealing their valuables and, in some cases, even their identities.

Some nursing homes will take anyone off the streets, it seems. What does this say about how they view their residents? Suppose your local fire department hired anyone who walked into the station—all without schooling or credentials, experience, or background checks—then paid them poorly? Such "firemen" might have to heed other impulses. How many arsonists would join the crew? Or thieves? How safe would you feel in your home?

Incensed by what I had found, I decided to return with microphone and camera crew to challenge the three homes who had hired me. Two refused to comment on camera either way. The owner of the third nursing home also declined an interview, though she did tell us this:

"We have a friend that we use to do our own background checks," she said. "We didn't use the bureau [OSBI] because we feel they are not thorough enough. We would rather rely on our own sources."

Their own sources? What could be more useful than the state's own criminal records? A credit check, perhaps? Perhaps next time she, too, should refuse to comment.

I asked the ex-convict whose identity I'd borrowed, "How safe would a resident of a nursing home be with you?"

At first he could only shake his head. Then his eyes narrowed. "It wouldn't have been safe at all for any of them," he said finally. "If I had . . .

I could get into a room, they were as good as if the devil had walked into the room himself."

Unthinkable, you still say? Hardly. The Justin Martins are out there. In many other cases, whole nursing-home staffs are to blame. The stories are everywhere, creating one vast and shocking tale.

REPORTS OF ABUSE, NEGLECT, AND CORRUPTION

Over a three-year span, Leslie Oliva moved her mother, Marie Espinoza, who had a degenerative brain disease, in and out of three California nursing homes. With every move Oliva thought she was taking her mother out of a bad situation into a better one. Instead, these three bleak years would prove to be the last of her mother's life.

Oliva's 1998 written statement to the Senate Special Committee on Aging said, in part, that within months of arriving at one convalescent hospital, her mother had bruises, bedsores, and a broken pelvis. Not only that, her mother began to lose weight, probably because food often was left out of her reach at the end of the bed. But Marie Espinoza's ordeal had just begun. She was moved to another nursing home and suffered severe dehydration and bedsores. Then she entered a third convalescent home. Marie Espinoza died, the nursing home reported, after choking on food. But that made little sense to her daughter. By that point, Espinoza was supposed to be fed through a tube. Still, all three nursing homes denied any wrongdoing.

The two-day hearing in July 1998 by the Senate Special Committee on Aging used a study by the General Accounting Office (GAO) as its foundation. The report, entitled "California Nursing Homes: Care Problems Persist Despite Federal and State Oversight," concluded that certain California nursing homes are not sufficiently monitored to guarantee the safety and welfare of their residents. This conclusion was based on data from federal surveys and state complaint investigations by the California Department of Health Services (DHS) on 1,370 California nursing homes.

Included in the report was a review of sixty-two records of residents who died in 1993 from fifteen randomly selected California nursing homes with at least five allegedly avoidable deaths per one hundred beds. The report found that residents in thirty-four cases had received unacceptable care. However, due to the lack of autopsy data, the GAO could not conclude whether or not this unacceptable care had contributed to the residents' deaths.

Between July 1995 and February 1998, out of the 1,370 nursing homes surveyed, 407, or almost 30 percent, were cited for serious deficiencies or potentially life-threatening care problems. In fact, *only 2 percent were found to have minimal or no deficiencies.* During the period from July 1995 to March 1998, one in eleven California nursing homes (122 homes), representing over 17,000 beds, were cited for conditions causing actual harm, putting residents in immediate jeopardy or causing death; federal sanctions were applied to only thirty-three of those homes.

The *national* compliance rate for the same period and for the same deficiencies was even worse: about one in nine homes, or 232,000 beds.

Listed below are some of the problems identified by the GAO report:

- One resident lost fifty-nine pounds, about a third of his body weight, over seven weeks. Until two days before he died, the staff had not recorded his weight since he had been admitted, nor did they notify a physician about his condition.
- Another resident who had five pressure sores, four that exposed the bone, was given pain medication only three times during five weeks of daily treatments to remove the dead tissue from her sores. She was unable to verbalize her needs and was reported to moan whenever this procedure was done without the pain medication.
- One resident, who was admitted to a home for physical-therapy rehabilitation after hip surgery, died five days later from septic shock caused by a urinary-tract infection. The staff had failed to monitor fluid intake and urine output after she was catheterized.

- Residents in one nursing home did not receive treatments, medications, or food supplements as ordered because the home lacked sufficient licensed nursing staff on duty.

The report also stated that the results only partially captured the extent of the care problems for the following reasons: homes are often able to predict the timing of annual reviews; medical staff can misrepresent the care provided; and deficiencies were missed due to methods used in the annual review.

Another problem uncovered during the California study was that the Health Care Financing Administration (HCFA), which oversees state agencies to ensure that nursing homes comply with federal standards and oversees the Medicare and Medicaid programs, didn't always ensure that homes were in substantial compliance before being reinstated. For example, a home was terminated on April 15, 1997, meaning that reimbursement for the home's Medicare and Medicaid beneficiaries stopped. After two surveys, the home was reinstated on June 1997. Because Medicare and Medicaid rules state that terminated nursing homes are to be paid for up to thirty days after termination, the home only lost three weeks of payment. Three months after reinstatement, DHS surveyors investigating a complaint found jeopardy violations due to a dangerously low number of staff; the home was also cited for substandard care when they found that some of the residents were left sitting in urine and feces for long periods of time and that residents were not getting proper care for urinary-tract infections.

The problems in California were not unique. Data from three reports presented in the committee's hearings in July 1998 and March 1999 showed that one-fourth of more than 17,000 nursing homes nationwide had serious deficiencies that caused harm to residents or placed them at risk of death or serious injury. Not only that, 40 percent of these homes had repeated serious deficiencies. According to statistics provided by the HCFA, 95 percent of nursing facilities remain open after receiving termination notices from the government.

During a question-and-answer period after a speech I'd given to law-enforcement agency managers, one nursing-home inspector from Kentucky said it was hard to shut down offending nursing homes because *there was no place to put the patients.*

So many reports, so many suffering patients. The federal government has promised a crackdown (I'll return to that). Isn't it about time?

ECONOMIC FRAUD IN NURSING HOMES

Another aspect to the nursing-home problem is economic fraud. In this scam, we're all victims. Whether against Medicare, Medicaid, or private insurers, economic fraud increases everyone's health care costs, much the same as shoplifting increases the costs of the food we eat and the clothes we wear.

I learned firsthand about fraudulent business practices while going undercover for the TV show *Inside Edition* as a freelance producer. Setting up an office complete with messy desk, file cabinets, stacks of folders and binders—and, of course, hidden cameras—I posed as a businessman about to open nursing homes in the area. Nursing-home patients need a lot of health care services, ranging from physical therapy to physician visits to wheelchairs. As the owner of the homes, I'd be able to pick and choose who provided those services.

I contacted several local health care service providers and invited them to my office to submit bids—to see just how far they would go to get at my share of Medicare patients. Most would go very far. More than half the companies offered some sort of kickback. Keep in mind here that it is a violation of federal law to either ask for or offer such kickbacks.

How big of a kickback? One supplier had this estimate: "I'd say, per claim, I might say $100 per patient." He ran a company providing physical therapy and home health services. Sitting at my desk, he had asked his female associate to leave my office before telling me just how much kickback—"referrals," some call them—he could offer. He had it all worked out.

"Let's say if we have thirty [patients] from you," he told me, "then thirty by a hundred dollars."

"Every two weeks?" I asked.

"Yes."

"Three thousand bucks every two weeks," I said, "six thousand bucks a month."

"We can, uh, work on that," he assured me. "Sure."

My take in his enormous Medicare profits would be six thousand bucks a month—and that was just his opening offer. Even then, it was just a drop in the bucket of the illicit money I could have pocketed. His company would provide only a fraction of the medical services my patients would be needing. His little office and mine—scamming Medicare together.

When confronted by my camera crew, he was at least honest. He told me that it's just business as usual. "It's unethical, I can tell you that," he said. "But you know, to get ahead in business, you have to scratch somebody's back."

To complicate matters, it's not always easy to tell a kickback from a harmless goodwill gift like a coffee mug. Where do you draw the line? That's what we asked a saleswoman from a national clinical laboratory which runs medical tests for patients across the country. The saleswoman met me in my office. With her happy, easygoing personality, she offered me the same questionable incentive she offers her big clients—in this case, $25 gift certificates.

I invited her back to a meeting room where she thought we'd be signing the deal. I had the papers in front of me. She smiled.

I recapped my understanding of her offer. "So, I can put anyone's name on here I want, including my own if I want to go out to dinner?" She nodded, smiled some more.

I nodded back and asked her to wait a moment—I'd be right back. Then in came fellow reporter Matt Meagher, microphone in hand and camera lights glaring behind him. Her smile dropped away.

"Aren't these gift certificates a giveaway?" he asked her.

She stood up. Her head was shaking now, and she stared at the table. "No, it is not," she muttered. "This is not a giveaway."

Not so fast—as it turned out, her bosses agreed with us. In a letter they claimed (while admitting the law is unclear on this area) that "our employee's conduct is in violation of [our company's] compliance policies . . ."

Kickbacks are one of the more pleasant ways of price-gouging. Smiles and scratched backs all around. But another way isn't so nice: providing services to people who simply don't need them.

One seventy-four-year-old nursing home resident on Medicare had trouble walking; she used a walker. She was told by rehabilitation experts that additional therapy would do her no good. Her bones were old, they said. Age does that to a person.

Still, a therapist from a local company said their expensive treatments could help her. Back in my pretend office, the company president told me how both our businesses could make extra money off patients. He said, "One way we can do it is, we can bill you and you bill them. We bill you at a lower rate, and you bill them at a higher rate." So, for example, they would bill us $80 for the useless treatments and we would bill Medicare $100, then pocket the difference.

He also offered me a $5,000 kickback if we let his company fill our prescriptions. They would also provide the services of their pharmacist for free. Not only that, they'd throw in a free computer! With that, I figured it was about time for the meeting room. We were in there, indicating that we were ready to sign. He had his coat off.

I clarified the offer: "So we get a pharmacist for free, five thousand bucks, and we get a computer?"

"Right," he assured me.

"Fine," I said. I stood, my finger at my chin. "Could you wait one moment? I'll be right back."

Out in the hallway, I called in the troops. But this company president wouldn't talk, and walked out. Our cameras followed, and we asked more questions. He strode down the hall and into the elevator, offering no comments on his way out.

The director of operations of a local ambulance company looked like a typical hospital administrator with his white shirt and tie and wire frame glasses when he stopped by. He wanted my nursing homes to refer all of our patients on kidney dialysis to his ambulance company.

"We'd like to know when you need something—like if you need a large-screen TV for your facility. We'd like to meet with someone at the administrative level and see if it's okay if we just present you with a complimentary funding check," he said. He went on to offer more large-screen TVs, stereos, even turkeys.

Turkeys and stereos, presents and perks. What does *any* of this have to do with health care services? Plenty. Good Medicare scams are so lucrative that those who operate them are willing to do what it takes and pay what it costs to secure them. And make no mistake—the money we're talking about is incredible. In 1999, the federal government estimated it would pay roughly $39 billion for nursing home care.

Back in my staged office, I leaned across the desk, looked the ambulance company representative in the eye, and asked, "You make how much on one dialysis patient?"

"Roughly around $360,000 a year," he replied again.

My eyes had stopped blinking. That's just for transporting one patient to and from a dialysis center. That's why some companies will do almost anything to collect Medicare patients.

"We make a lot of money," he had assured me.

It didn't take long to figure out why. With our hidden cameras, we taped one dialysis patient walking unaccompanied to one of his company's ambulances. A soft hold on the patient's arm helped him into the back, and he was off to the dialysis center. In an ambulance.

Did he really need an ambulance? That's hard to know for sure. But a cab would have cost $8.10 each way. This company charges Medicare up to $600 *each way*.

The Department of Health and Human Services (DHHS) Office of the Inspector General's study, "Physical and Occupational Therapy in Nursing Homes: Quality of Care and Medical Necessity for Medicare

Patients," found that almost 13 percent of therapy was improperly billed to Medicare because it was not medically necessary or was provided by inappropriate staff. The study looked at the physical and occupational therapy of a random sample of 218 Medicare patients in March 1998. In another report by the Inspector General, it is estimated that for the twelve-month period ending June 30, 1998, nursing facilities were paid almost $1 billion for improperly billed therapy and $331 million for improperly documented therapy. Because the facilities charged Medicare significantly more than they paid for occupational therapy, the cost of this markup to Medicare was estimated at $342 million a year.

EFFORTS TO IMPROVE STANDARDS

As demonstrated in a series of reports about California nursing homes presented to the Senate Special Committee on Aging, complaints alleging serious care problems were not being investigated and even when deficiencies were identified, state and federal policies were not effective in ensuring that these deficiencies were corrected. Moreover, the methods used by the state surveys, such as time spent and number of residents to review, are inconsistent.

Since the 1998 hearings the HCFA has been implementing initiatives to strengthen efforts to ensure the quality of care of the nearly 1.6 million Americans in the nation's nursing homes. Some of the initiatives include:

- **Improved survey processes used by states,** including a more rapid response time to complaints alleging harm to residents and revision of inspection times to include weekends and evenings.
- **Stricter enforcement to ensure nursing homes comply with federal requirements.** The states will be required to conduct more revisits to ensure serious deficiencies are corrected and those homes with poor compliance records will be inspected more frequently.
- **A revision of the definition of homes categorized as "poorly performing."** The homes with deficiencies would then be subject to immediate

sanctions. (Current policy allows for a grace period, generally thirty to sixty days, to correct deficiencies.)

- **Expansion of monetary penalties** so that homes are fined not only per day but on a per-instance basis.
- **Reevaluating policies related to terminated homes.** The new standards will: ensure that federal payments are made to terminated homes only if they are actively transferring residents to other locations; provide guidance on the appropriate length of time in which a home shows it has eliminated deficiencies before it can participate in the Medicare program; and ensure that the home's pre-termination compliance history is considered in subsequent enforcement actions after it has been readmitted to Medicare.
- **Better consumer access to information** about homes' compliance and quality of care. Already there are Internet sites set up with this information.
- States have been directed by the HCFA to impose **immediate sanctions against nursing homes for each serious incident that has threatened a resident's health or safety;** the facilities can be fined up to $10,000 for each incident.
- States are required to make **more frequent inspections of those nursing homes with a record of abuse.** They also have the flexibility to stop payments for new admissions to these nursing homes.

Is the crackdown working? After the HCFA's policy letter recommending that complaints alleging harm to residents be investigated within ten workdays, some states responded by saying they required additional personnel. But even so, some nursing homes are getting caught and punished. A recent spate of multimillion-dollar jury awards to nursing-home residents and their families may, hopefully, force such facilities to improve.

As reported by the Georgia State Health Care Fraud Control Unit in Leslie Aronovitz's November 9, 1999, testimony to the House of Representatives Subcommittee on Oversight and Investigations, two

businessmen were involved in a complex scheme of submitting fraudulent nursing-home cost reports to the Medicaid program. Through their
nursing-home chain and shell corporation, they billed Medicaid for
inflated expenses related to phony contracts with the nursing home.
Their scheme made them nearly $10 million. One defendant received
fifty months in prison and a $70,000 fine; his partner got a thirty-six month
prison sentence and a $50,000 fine. They both received another three
years of supervised release. As restitution, the pair agreed to pay about $6
million to the state Medicaid program.

In August 1999 it was announced that the nation's largest nursing-
home chain, Beverly Enterprises, agreed to pay $175 million and remove
ten of its nursing homes from the Medicare and Medicaid programs in
order to settle pending criminal and civil cases filed against it by the federal government. The government alleges that the Fort Smith, Arizona,
company overbilled Medicare for nursing labor costs from 1990 to 1997.
Beverly operates 563 skilled nursing facilities and hundreds of other
long-term care facilities, including assisted-living centers and home
health agencies.

Remember what the first unscrupulous supplier told me about
"business as usual"? Sounds like the same old drill. And, with as many
nursing homes as there are out there, you have to wonder how many are
still going about business as usual for every one that gets caught.

CHOOSING A NURSING HOME

Before you begin to look into nursing homes, first determine what level
of care is needed. There are a variety of options, such as home and community services (Meals on Wheels), assisted living for those who don't
require medical care, board and care homes, and retirement communities And be sure to talk to people you trust, such as family, friends, and
perhaps health professionals who understand your needs.

There is a wealth of information about nursing homes available
through the governmental agencies, such as the DHHS's Office of the

Inspector General, HCFA, Medicare, and the Administration on Aging, and private organizations such as Healthgrades and the Association for the Protection of the Elderly. (I've listed these contacts and others in the appendix.) Many of these organizations give information about Medicare- and Medicaid-certified nursing homes, including location, availability, staffing, quality of care, and results from their latest inspection. You can also seek help through the Long-Term Care Ombudsmen program in your state. These programs, which are administered by the Administration on Aging, have thousands of trained volunteer ombudsmen who regularly visit long-term care facilities and monitor their conditions and care.

Contact the Health Department or Better Business Bureau in your area. See if complaints have been filed against the facility, and if the home submits background checks on its employees. Ask for references and talk to residents and employees.

Visit the nursing home more than once. The first time you visit, you will probably be given a formal tour. After the tour, find different times and days when you can return for a visit. Ask to see a copy of the home's most recent inspection; by law, the report must be posted in an area where residents and visitors can view it. The HCFA's booklet *Your Guide to Choosing a Nursing Home* has a checklist that will help you evaluate the nursing homes you visit on things such as facts about the nursing home and its staff, quality of life, quality of care, and nutrition and hydration. Remember that quality care comes from quality people, so check out the staff carefully.

After you narrow your list of choices, conduct follow-up visits. Be sure that you visit at least once during a weekend and in the evening to observe staffing and care giving. If you are able, try to attend a meeting of the nursing home's resident or family council, which is involved in the quality of life for the residents, and stay for a meal. Look for any unreasonable use of restraints on patients. Observe the facility for cleanliness and odor. Also, get a copy of the admission contract or agreement and read it carefully. If you still have any questions, contact an Ombudsman volunteer. Have an attorney review the nursing-home contract before you or a loved one signs anything.

WHAT YOU CAN DO TO FIGHT FRAUD AND/OR ABUSE

First and foremost, frequent contact with those in the outside world is *critical*. If no one visits, how can the treatment of a resident be evaluated?

If you or someone close to you is already in a nursing home, remember that nursing-home residents and their relatives and friends have rights and special protections under the law. If you think your rights or those of your loved one are being violated, express your concerns to someone on the staff if you feel comfortable doing so. For a serious concern, you might want to file a complaint with the state's inspection agency. Do keep in mind that response times vary from state to state. If your problem isn't resolved to your satisfaction, start looking for a new home.

If you suspect abuse, *make that call*. It could be a matter of life or death.

chapter 12

Shopping for Supplements

Buying a Pig in a Poke

PICTURE THIS: I'M WEARING my trusty white lab coat in the middle of a Houston shopping mall. A stethoscope is draped around my neck. To my left is a sign that reads "All Natural Steroid" and shows a heavily muscled male arm. Another sign asks, "Are You Really Potent?" Behind me is a third sign that advertises an "All Natural Baldness Cure." Stacks of testimonials and other promotional literature surround me on a simple table flanked by folding chairs. Anyone approaching will hear me proclaim that my new products will overcome potency problems and baldness. I also claim that my natural steroids will increase strength and build muscle. On our undercover videotape you can hear me tell a potential customer that with Flex2000, a fifteen-minute workout would equal four hours of exercise.

If you think that no one would ever swallow such preposterous tales, think again.

In reality, I was pretending to be *"Dr."* Chuck Whitlock for a television show. We'd placed professional-looking labels on bottles of plain vitamin C tablets to see who'd fall for my outrageous claims about three fictitious dietary supplements. No one was more surprised at the outcome than I was.

One after another, individuals readily parted with their cash. Few of them asked any questions. I even convinced a popular minor-league hockey player to buy my Flex2000 pills after listening to him describe his physically grueling schedule.

I told one balding gentleman that a year ago my hair had looked about the way his did—before I started using our creation called HairTech. He replied, "Hey, if this works, I'll be a distributor for you."

When I told him that our company could use a distributor in the Houston area, he shocked me when he responded, "I can go anywhere in the world. I'm a physician." After he paid cash for a bottle, I asked him if he was going to buy stock in my company after the product worked for him in thirty days. He retorted, "I'll buy you out!"

Of course, I gave all the buyers their money back and let them know what I was really doing. I asked why they were so willing to buy pills with such outlandish claims from a total stranger. The real doctor probably summed it up best: "Everybody's looking for the dream come true."

WHAT EXACTLY ARE "DIETARY SUPPLEMENTS"— and Who Needs Them, Anyway?

According to the FDA, surveys show that more than 50 percent of adult Americans use dietary supplements. Sales of such products were projected to skyrocket to a whopping $15.7 billion for the year 2000, according to the *Nutrition Business Journal*.

Since supplements are freely available without a prescription, they're easy to get. And the ready availability of such products creates the widespread assumption that they are always safe and wholesome. This assumption, however, is a myth. Using supplements carelessly or without the right information can result in serious illness or even death.

The National Institutes of Health's Office of Dietary Supplements (ODS) defines a dietary supplement as

> . . . a product (other than tobacco) intended to supplement the
> diet that bears or contains one or more of the following dietary

ingredients: a vitamin, mineral, amino acid, herb, or other botanical; OR a dietary substance for use to supplement the diet by increasing the total dietary intake; OR a concentrate, metabolite, constituent, extract, or combination of any ingredient described above; AND intended for ingestion in the form of a capsule, powder, softgel, or gelcap, and not represented as a conventional food or as a sole item of a meal or the diet.

What a mouthful.

The bottom line is that dietary supplements are distinct from drugs, which are intended to diagnose, cure, mitigate, treat, or prevent diseases. Historically the most common type of dietary supplement in the United States has been a multivitamin/mineral tablet. In a survey of 33,905 Americans published in the March 2000 issue of *Archives of Family Medicine,* 40 percent of the respondents reported taking at least one vitamin or mineral supplement during a previous month.

Although many medical practitioners and nutritionists agree that healthy adults can get the necessary nutrients from a well-balanced diet, how many of us regularly eat properly? According to the Mayo Clinic Health Oasis Web site, it's estimated that only one in ten Americans regularly eats the five servings of fruits and vegetables recommended for good nutrition. Repeated surveys of clinical nutritionists have found that even a high percentage of these professionals feel the need to add supplements to their own diets. And if you are elderly, smoke, are on a restricted diet, drink alcohol excessively, or are pregnant, breast-feeding, or chronically ill, you especially need to talk to your doctor about what, if any, supplements you might need.

On the Quackwatch Web site, consumer advocates Stephen Barrett, M.D., and Victor Herbert, M.D., J.D., warn that some vitamin pushers pitch supplements as "insurance" against vitamin deficiency. These promoters typically claim that most diseases are due to poor nutrition, or tell you that "all-natural" vitamins are superior to synthetic ones so you'll buy their products. Barrett and Herbert warn of unscientific practitioners who utilize bogus tests like hair analysis to determine exactly what your body's nutritional needs are and—does this surprise you?—which of their products you should purchase to rectify the problems that they are all but certain to find. Naturally there will be something "special" about their supplements that sets them apart from, and makes them considerably more expensive than, the inexpensive generic supplements available at your local discount drugstore.

When researching this chapter, I searched the Internet for general information about vitamin E. To my amazement, I found a staggering 3,900-plus listings on Yahoo Shopping alone for vitamin E. But covering the pros and cons of every vitamin, mineral, and herbal product out there is beyond the scope of this book. Instead, my objective is to give you enough general information about supplements that you'll do your own investigation before you start swallowing megadoses of vitamin C or St. John's wort just because someone told you that it will make you healthier or happier. Contrary to popular belief, many supplements do have a downside. As with drugs, the very characteristics that make a supplement desirable under one set of circumstances may make it totally detrimental to your health under another. Keep in mind here that the only way a supplement can be "totally safe" under all circumstances is if it is totally ineffective under *any* circumstances.

Efficacy is also an important consideration about supplements. Do they really do what they're supposed to? A recent study by the U.S. Department of Agriculture (USDA) examined forty-six commercial preparations touted to be "strong antioxidants." The chief scientific agency of the USDA tested supplements containing bilberry, cranberry, chokeberry, elderberry, grape seed, and pine bark extracts. Their findings? That a day's suggested dosage of twenty-nine of the forty-six products tested wouldn't provide as much antioxidant capacity as a single serving of fruits or vegetables. Since there are no industry standards for the antioxidant capacity of natural product supplements, there's little assurance of getting an effective, quality product.

How do you know if a supplement is safe and effective for you? What supplements should you avoid? What are the tip-offs that you're being ripped off by a MediScammer? Let's take a look.

THE POTENTIAL DANGERS OF SUPPLEMENTS

When taking supplements the two immediate concerns you should have are that they may be toxic or contaminated. "Toxicity" refers to the inherent poisonous or otherwise negative effects that may result from taking a supplement. Just about any substance can be toxic if it's consumed in sufficient quantities, even vitamins. For example, high dosages of vitamin A over a period of time can cause liver damage, bone damage, and may result in birth defects if taken during pregnancy. Bone deformity and kidney damage can result from overdosing on vitamin D. And just because something's "natural" doesn't mean it's safe. That's why it's crucial to heed all the warnings on a supplement's label—assuming, of course, that the known dangers are even mentioned there in the first place.

The television segment in which I sold bogus products in the middle of a shopping mall was only one of several I've done on dietary supplements. For another television segment, I investigated whether dietary supplements really contain the ingredients in the exact amounts the labels claim they do. Several of the manufacturers we interviewed produced the supplement creatine, which advocates say enhances athletic performance. When reporters disclosed that baseball superstars Sammy Sosa and Mark McGwire used creatine, why shouldn't the next generation of up-and-coming athletes try it to get a competitive edge? If it can improve athletic performance while decreasing fatigue as its proponents claim, what's the harm? That's a good question. Unfortunately, the answer isn't one that athletes who take such supplements want to hear.

McGwire also admitted he'd taken "andro," the hormone androstenedione, another supposed performance-enhancing substance that marketers claim increases testosterone. In fact, in February 2000 a Major League Baseball–funded study found that andro (which is banned by the National Football League, the Olympics, and the National Collegiate Athletic Association) does indeed raise testosterone levels. But that's not really good news. Artificially increased testosterone levels are associated with acne, liver and heart damage, and personality disorders. No wonder the Major League Baseball study concluded that taking "andro" could be hazardous to your health. Despite the testimonials, there isn't any hard evidence that either creatine or andro enhances athletic performance as claimed.

"Contamination" refers to impurities introduced during the manufacturing process. While reports of contamination of supplements are somewhat rare, the results can still be tragic. In 1989 a contaminant in tryptophan supplements from Japan caused an outbreak of eosinophilia-myalgia syndrome (EMS), a rare disorder that reportedly killed forty Americans and injured some one thousand more. Almost ten years later, six brands of the tryptophan derivative 5-HTP (5 hydroxy-L-tryptophan) sold in nutrition stores were found to contain levels of a contaminant called "peak x," which researchers believe could result in EMS.

THE PRINCIPLE PROPONENTS OF SUPPLEMENTS—
Complementary and Alternative Medicine Practitioners

Alternative medicine has a growing number of followers not only in the United States but throughout the industrialized world. In Germany and France, physicians routinely prescribe herbal and homeopathic medicines. In the United Kingdom, homeopathy has long enjoyed a measure of popularity. The AMA estimates that, worldwide, up to 90 percent of all health care is what we would consider "alternative."

The Complementary and Alternative Health Care Freedom of Access Act was signed into law in May 2000 in Minnesota. The first of its kind in the United States, the law enables Minnesota alternative health care practitioners to practice without fear of being charged with practicing medicine without a license. The Department of Health will oversee the practitioners and investigate all consumer complaints. The law does not establish credential or training requirements to determine which kinds of healing are legitimate and which aren't. The law is effective July 2001.

Proponents of complementary health care state that the law recognizes their right to practice, while the law's critics are concerned that it will legitimize even the wackiest ideas. Bob McCoy, curator of the Museum of Questionable Medical Devices located in Minneapolis, told the *Star Tribune* that the law "makes about two-thirds of the things in our museum now legitimate."

The list of alternative therapies is extensive—it includes acupuncture, aromatherapy, biofeedback, chiropractic, colonic irrigation, holistic health, homeopathy, hypnotherapy, light therapy, magnetic-field therapy, naturopathic medicine, osteopathic medicine, reflexology, and therapeutic touch, just to name a few of the better-known ones. Over time, aspects of some of these therapies have become more accepted by conventional medicine than others.

Frequently, alternative therapies involve an entire philosophy or belief system. For example, holistic health is based upon the belief that a person should strive not just to be free of disease but to achieve wellness. This can be achieved only by balancing the physical, emotional, mental, and spiritual aspects of an individual. Advocates believe that within each of us is the power to create that wellness—the power of choice. They believe that a person's health is his own responsibility.

Naturopathic medicine is a form of holistic medicine. It embraces a philosophical approach to health that relies upon natural, noninvasive remedies. Naturopaths claim to treat the whole person, using the person's own natural ability to heal himself. Although naturopathic physicians use the title "doctor," they are not licensed or regulated in most states, and they cannot prescribe drugs or perform surgery. As with most holistic practitioners, their diagnoses and suggested treatments rely heavily upon the patient's diet and lifestyle.

Some naturopathic recommendations such as natural childbirth and acupuncture have developed a following among consumers and many conventional physicians alike. Many of its dietary tenets, such as a diet high in fruits, vegetables, and whole grains, have become standard prescriptions for a healthy lifestyle. Other naturopathic recommendations, such as the use of homeopathic medicines, fasting, and "detoxifying" enemas, have little or no scientific foundation. Naturopaths typically recommend the use of vitamins, minerals, enzymes, "natural" hormone preparations, and whole herbs or extracts as opposed to synthetic medications. Among the dangers of treating diseases with dietary supplements is that the potency of the products used by naturopaths is usually not standardized, so it can vary widely.

Homeopathy, another holistic approach, was addressed earlier in chapter 10, "Potent or Placebo?" Homeopathy's founder, Samuel Hahnemann, believed that disease represented a disturbance in the body's ability to heal itself. His "law of similars" resulted in the creation of homeopathic remedies made from mixing water or alcohol with herbs, minerals, and other substances, as we discussed earlier. The FDA does not check homeopathic products for safety or effectiveness (more on the FDA's role in the next section). However, acting out of concern that unlicensed, untrained homeopathic practitioners were treating patients for serious illnesses, the FDA mandated in 1988 that "homeopathic drugs cannot be offered without prescription for such serious conditions as cancer, AIDS, or any other requiring diagnosis and treatment by a licensed practitioner. Nonprescription homeopathics may be sold only for self-limiting conditions recognizable by consumers." In other words, over-the-counter homeopathic preparations only can be sold to treat conditions that should go away on their own.

Another important consideration is that some supplements can interact with certain drugs in detrimental ways. For example, though its proponents insist that ginkgo biloba improves circulation, memory, and mental function, the herb has also been shown to contribute to the anticoagulant effect of aspirin and other drugs, which could lead to bleeding.

And because herbs aren't as well-regulated as other supplements, they are subject to being misidentified, contaminated, or mixed with other ingredients that might be harmful.

The direst consequence of relying only on alternative therapies is the possibility that a serious medical problem could go undiagnosed and untreated by proven conventional methods. Responsible naturopathic and homeopathic practitioners will refer serious, urgent, and potentially life-threatening cases to a qualified medical specialist. The problem here is that practitioners who are not trained in conventional medicine must be relied upon to recognize conditions that require conventional medical treatment and make the appropriate referral. Even the most well-intentioned alternative-medicine practitioner might not recognize the early signs of a serious medical emergency.

A HAMSTRUNG FDA OFFERS ONLY LIMITED PROTECTION

On a hot Southern California day in April 1998, a healthy twenty-seven-year-old man took a drink from a water bottle his friend had set on a table. He had taken a few chugs before realizing the clear liquid wasn't water. By then it was too late. The bottle contained gamma hydroxybutyrate (GHB), a party drug so popular at clubs that some kids still consider it an alternative to drinking alcohol. At the time no one was overly concerned about the young man drinking the mixture, and friends just told his roommate to check on him every so often to make sure he was still breathing. His friends got an abrupt wake-up call when he unexpectedly died.

First synthesized in 1960, GHB was sold in health food stores as a dietary supplement. It became popular among bodybuilders in the 1980s because it supposedly caused the body to release a growth hormone and stimulate muscle growth. GHB has powerful side effects including nausea, vomiting, delusions, depression, vertigo, hallucinations, seizures, difficulty breathing, decreased heart rate, low blood pressure, amnesia, and coma. It has never been approved for sale as a medical product in the U.S.

Since 1990 the FDA has issued numerous warnings to consumers about the potentially lethal side effects of GHB and its chemical "cousins," gamma butyrolactone (GBL) and 1,4 butanediol (BD). Congress has since outlawed as dangerous drugs GHB and precursors that metabolize to GHB inside the human body. Guy Gugliotta reported in the *Washington Post* that the Drug Enforcement Administration (DEA) had officially listed sixty deaths associated with GHB-type supplements across the country.

We'd all like to think the government is able to protect us, and that the FDA wouldn't allow unsafe products to be sold in the U.S. at all—least of all in health food stores. But unlike prescription and over-the-counter medications, supplements are relatively free of government regulation due to the Dietary Supplement and Health Education Act of 1994 (DSHEA). The result is that the FDA doesn't test or approve dietary supplements before they're marketed. Thanks to DSHEA, the FDA can only take action against a supplement if it poses an unreasonable health risk or is being sold as a drug.

Citing the lack of comprehensive statistics for tracking the incidence of sickness and death associated with supplements, the *Washington Post* article published the findings of its first nationwide survey of health officials, researchers, and advocates about dietary supplements. While admitting that it was impossible to compare individual studies, given that the various researchers gathered their information in different ways, among the *Post*'s discoveries were that:

- Dangerous contaminants continue to be found in supplements. In 1998 California investigators found that almost 33 percent of the 260 imported Asian herbal supplements they investigated contained toxic compounds such as lead, arsenic, mercury, or extraneous drugs that were not disclosed on the label copy.
- A growing number of children are victims of supplement abuse. This is important because even children's vitamins that have been supplemented with iron can be toxic when children take more than the recommended dosage.

- Poison control centers around the country are reporting adverse reactions to a broad range of supplements including ginseng, St. John's wort, ephedra, and melatonin.
- Individual states receive far more reports of adverse reactions to supplements than does the FDA. Even so, the FDA reported 2,621 adverse events including 184 deaths—involving supplements between 1993 and 1998. By contrast, the American Association of Poison Control Centers received 6,914 reports of toxic reactions to supplements in 1998 alone, and almost 1,400 of these required that the victim be treated in a health care facility. To add to the confusion, the numbers from the Poison Control Centers don't include reports about ephedrine or its derivatives, which account for the greatest number of the FDA's adverse-events reports.

Further, in 1999, one San Francisco trial lawyer deposed an executive of a company whose ephedrine-based product had generated an estimated 3,500 complaints, none of which were reported to the FDA. Clearly the adverse reactions to food supplements are underreported and underestimated.

Although manufacturers and distributors don't need to register with the FDA or get its approval before producing or selling dietary supplements, the manufacturer is responsible for ensuring that label information is truthful and not misleading to consumers. The manufacturer is also responsible for ensuring that this list of ingredients is accurate, that the ingredients are safe, and that the product's content matches what's on the label. In theory, that's the way everyone is supposed to do it—all the supplement manufacturers monitor themselves and protect public safety. And if you think it really works that way, you haven't been reading this book very carefully.

Due to its limited resources, the FDA rarely steps in unless there's a public health emergency where supplements have been directly implicated in injury, illness, or death. In the wake of the withdrawal from the market of the drugs fenfluramine (marketed as Pondimin) and dexfenfluramine (marketed as Redux) following the 1997 fen-phen scare (discussed in chapter 6), the FDA also issued public warnings about *herbal* fen-phen products. The FDA considered such products to be unapproved drugs because they were promoted as alternatives to the anti-obesity drugs. Of course, an "FDA Warning" is only as good as the FDA's ability to get the word out to individual consumers and the consumers' willingness to comply with the advice.

The FDA's next priority when it comes to dietary supplements is analyzing products thought to be fraudulent or illegal. Remember, though, that the FDA doesn't analyze dietary supplements *before* they're sold to consumers. For all practical purposes, that means that a supplement not only must be already on the store shelves but generating consumer complaints before the FDA even takes a look at it. And once a supplement is on the market, the FDA must show that it is unsafe before taking action to restrict the product's use.

What does this really mean? *That we, the consumers, share responsibility with the supplement manufacturers for determining the safety of a dietary supplement and the veracity of the claims made on its label.*

In November 1999 the FDA warned the public about taking Triax Metabolic Accelerator, which was being sold as a dietary supplement for those wanting to lose weight. The agency had determined that it was actually a *new, unapproved drug* containing a potent thyroid hormone that could lead to heart attacks and strokes. The FDA learned about the product through its MedWatch reporting system, which had received reports of individuals who'd experienced severe diarrhea, fatigue, lethargy, or profound weight loss while taking the supplement. The FDA not only issued a consumer warning, but got the state of Missouri, where the product's principle distributor was located, to embargo the product. The FDA also got a voluntary agreement from the manufacturer to stop distributing it.

But the need for consumer vigilance never ends. As this was being written, a company was advertising over the Internet a supplement which it claimed to be an identical product to Triax Metabolic Accelerator.

Consumers can report an adverse event or illness they think is related to a dietary supplement by calling the FDA at 1-800-FDA-1088 or by using the Web site http://www.fda.gov/medwatch/report/consumer/consumer.htm. You can also report problems through FDA district offices across the country.

SOME PROBLEM SUPPLEMENTS

According to the FDA, most vitamin and mineral supplements are normally safe for the general population. What most concerns the FDA in the area of dietary supplements is the vast array of other nutritional products, such as amino acids, herbs, and other botanicals, whose safety and efficacy is unsubstantiated. The amount of the various natural constituents in herbal supplements can vary substantially depending upon the part of the plant it comes from, where it was in its growth stage when it was harvested, as well as various elements of the manufacturing process. Substances in dietary supplements that have raised safety issues include the following:

- **Chaparral (herb).** Promoters have claimed it slows aging and cleanses the blood, but the FDA has warned consumers of possibly irreversible liver disease.
- **Comfrey (herb).** Sold as teas, tablets, capsules, tinctures, poultices, and lotions, comfrey may obstruct blood flow to the liver, in some cases resulting in death.
- **Germanium (mineral).** Thought by some to have antioxidant properties, long-term use of this nonessential element may cause serious, irreversible kidney damage or death.
- **Guar gum (complex carbohydrate).** Commonly used as a food thickener, this product can cause diarrhea, vomiting, bloating, and intestinal blockage. It's been used in weight loss products to produce a feeling of fullness, but one brand sent ten users to the hospital and one to the morgue following surgery to remove a throat blockage. It's been banned from use as an active ingredient in over the-counter weight loss products.

- **Ephedra (herb).** Also called ma huang or epitonin, it is a major source of the stimulant ephedrine, as discussed earlier in this chapter. Commonly used in products designed to control weight and boost energy, this herb has been reported to produce high blood pressure, rapid or irregular heart rate, nerve damage, muscle injury, insomnia, psychosis, heart attack, stroke, and death.
- **Yohimbe (herb).** Marketed in bodybuilding and "enhanced male performance" products, this tree bark has been linked to kidney failure, seizures, and death.
- **DHEA (hormone).** Advocates of this hormone claim it fights aging, but it could increase the risk of cancer and liver damage even if taken only briefly.
- **"Dieter's teas" (herbal blends).** These typically contain such laxatives as senna *(Cassia angustifolia),* aloe, rhubarb root, buckthorn, cascara, and castor oil. Use of these teas can lead to nausea, diarrhea, vomiting, stomach cramps, chronic constipation, fainting, or even death.
- **Pennyroyal (herb).** A member of the mint family, it is used to induce abortion. It can produce severe bleeding and is responsible for at least one death.
- **Sassafras (herb).** Because the oil from this plant has been shown to cause liver cancer in animals, it has been banned as a food additive in the U.S. The herb is still sold as a supplement for tonics and teas.
- **Lobelia (herb).** Also known as Indian tobacco, it contains lobeline, which has been used to treat asthma and other respiratory symptoms, including those of colds and flu. Low doses may result in breathing problems, while higher doses may bring on a rapid heartbeat, low blood pressure, coma, or death.

THE DANGERS OF EXCESSIVE POTENCY

Excessive potency of certain ingredients may also cause adverse effects. For example, the FDA ordered some calcium supplements reformulated after discovering that they contained too much vitamin D. Although the margin between what's safe and necessary and what's toxic is very large for some nutrients, for others this margin is very small. Some known risks of nutrients taken at excessive potencies follow.

- **Folic acid.** Taking more than 1 milligram per day can disguise a vitamin B12 deficiency.
- **Iron.** Vitamins containing iron are an all-too-common cause of U.S. child poisoning deaths. High dosages in adults have been linked to heart disease.
- **Niacin.** High intakes can cause liver damage, severe gastrointestinal problems, eye damage, muscle disease, and damage to the heart.
- **Selenium.** High intakes for even a few weeks can damage the body's tissues.
- **Vitamin A.** Continuous high intakes can cause headaches, liver damage, bone damage, diarrhea, and birth defects.
- **Vitamin B6.** High intakes are linked to bone pain, muscle weakness, balance problems, numbness, and other nerve-disorder symptoms.
- **Vitamin C.** Although proponents of high intakes of vitamin C tout its greatness, diarrhea and urinary-tract problems such as kidney stones may result when consumed at excessive doses.
- **Vitamin D.** Bone deformity and kidney damage may result from regular ingestion of high doses.

SUPPLEMENT-DRUG INTERACTIONS

One of the most potentially dangerous, yet underreported, aspects of supplement usage is that some supplements interact with prescription medications. To make matters worse, someone taking supplements may not even associate a side effect or negative reaction with the supplement, especially if they're taking other medications or if they're chronically ill. Some adverse effects take time to develop and present themselves, so a consumer may not even consider the possibility that a supplement he's taking may be the culprit. Licorice, flaxseed, kava kava, bromelain, and high doses of vitamin E have been known to interact dangerously with prescription medications.

When your physician routinely asks you what medications are you taking, do you mention any vitamins, herbal teas, or other supplements you might regularly ingest? According to a Mayo Clinic study, almost two-thirds of people taking herbal supplements don't tell their health care providers what they're taking. It's important that physicians specifically ask about supplements, and that consumers know exactly what they're taking and volunteer this information even when the physician forgets to ask about it. Consider the following two advisories:

On February 10, 2000, the FDA issued a public health advisory concerning the herbal product St. John's wort *(Hypericum perforatum)*. A study by the National Institutes of Health revealed significant interaction between the supplement and indinavir, a protease inhibitor used to treat HIV. Based on this study the FDA stated that the herbal supplement might significantly decrease blood concentrations of all the currently marketed HIV protease inhibitors, and might also have the same effect on certain other drugs.

California's State Health Director, Diana Bont, R.N., Dr. P. H., issued another consumer alert on February 15, 2000. According to this alert, "consumers should immediately stop using five herbal products because they contain two prescription drugs not listed as ingredients that are unsafe without monitoring by a physician." The five products in question were Diabetes Hypoglucose Capsules, Pearl Hypoglycemic Capsules, Tongyi Tang Diabetes Angel Pearl Hypoglycemic Capsules, Tongyi Tang Diabetes Angel Hypoglycemic Capsules, and Zen Qi Capsules. Although the products claimed to contain only natural Chinese herbal ingredients, the investigation by the California DHS determined they contained glyburide and phenformin, two prescription drugs used to treat diabetes.

Just two months later, Diabetic Capital recalled its product Dianolyn Capsules, and SciQuest Lab, Inc., recalled Dimelstat, both supplements said to contain glyburide in dangerously high amounts.

NEW LABELING REQUIREMENTS LIMIT CLAIMS

In January 2000 the FDA issued its new rules limiting what claims dietary supplements may make. Such products may make claims relating to the effects that they have on the structure or function of the body ("structure/function claims") without prior FDA review. Acceptable claims would include "maintains a healthy circulatory system," or "for common symptoms of PMS." They may not, however, bear an express or implied claim that they can prevent, treat, cure, mitigate, or diagnose disease without prior FDA review. (This is called a "disease claim".) An example of a prohibited disease claim would be "prevents osteoporosis" or "lowers cholesterol."

This doesn't mean, however, that every supplement you purchase right away will be in compliance with the new requirements. The FDA gave small businesses that marketed a product as of January 6, 2000, an additional seventeen months to bring existing claims into compliance. Other dietary supplements already on the market have an additional eleven months to be in compliance.

THE FTC—Advertising's Arthritic Watchdog

While the FDA governs claims made for dietary supplements on labels, package inserts, and other materials presented at the point of sale, the FTC is charged with regulating the *advertising* claims of such products. Its "truth in advertising" law is intended to mandate that advertising claims for dietary supplements be truthful, not misleading, and substantiated with reliable scientific evidence.

The FTC's stated philosophy is that the overall image of the product set forth in the ad is important. What the FTC considers is the general impression a consumer gets, and whether it's truthful. Both express and implied claims are to be considered. For example, if an ad claims that 90 percent of all cardiologists regularly take the dietary supplement being advertised, the implication is that the product offers some benefit for the heart. In this case, the advertiser is supposed to be able to support both the express claims (90 percent of cardiologists take the product) as well as the implied claim (the supplement benefits the heart).

The FTC also demands—in theory, anyway—that all health-related claims be backed up by scientific evidence. Opinions and real-life experiences, even if true, aren't enough. And while testimonials are permitted, if that person's results are not typical, a disclaimer to that effect is supposed to accompany the testimonial. For example, if someone lost thirty-five pounds while taking a weight loss product but also exercised and dieted at the same time, this is supposed to be prominently disclosed. Also, research would have to show that the product contributed to the weight loss beyond what would be produced by diet and exercise alone.

In theory the FTC protects us against bogus or misleading advertising claims made by supplement manufacturers. But how effective is the agency in living up to its own mission? In March 1999 the FTC charged that the claims made by Rose Creek Health Products, Inc., for the dietary supplement "Vitamin O" were false and that the substance appeared to contain little more than salt water. The FTC filed an injunction against the company and its sister corporation, The Staff of Life, Inc., citing their ads claimed the supplement could prevent or cure cancer, heart disease, and lung disease. Scientists said there was no scientific basis for those claims, and nutrition experts do not recognize the existence of a "vitamin O."

The FTC's complaint quotes statements made by Rose Creek in an ad in *USA Today:* ". . . 'Vitamin O' has helped eliminate everything from breathing problems and lack of energy to life-threatening diseases." An Internet ad quoted in the complaint contained glowing testimonials, such as the following:

> My father had . . . open-heart surgery. . . . One of the common side effects is absolutely excruciating leg pains . . . He took just 30 drops of 'Vitamin O' orally twice a day, and in two days the pain disappeared! . . . It has also provided very significant relief for his emphysema.

Rose Creek, which reported selling nearly a million bottles of the supplement for up to $25 each, responded by saying its customers get more than salt water—they get stabilized oxygen. According to the FTC's complaint, the company's ads identify the contents of "Vitamin O" as "intact oxygen molecules in a liquid solution of distilled water, sodium chloride, and trace minerals." This is the kind of nonsensical pseudoscientific gibberish that MediScammers typically use to confuse and impress whomever they're trying to swindle.

On May 1, 2000, the FTC announced that the marketers of "Vitamin O" had agreed to pay $375,000 to settle the agency's charges that their claims were false and unsubstantiated. As noted earlier, a consent decree is for settlement purposes only and doesn't constitute an admission of a law violation.

So, how successful was the FTC campaign against "Vitamin O"? More than two weeks after the FTC announced its settlement with the marketers of "Vitamin O," a product referred to as "Stabilized Oxygen" was still being advertised on the Internet. Promoters said that, due to FDA restrictions, "Stabilized Oxygen" had replaced the name "Vitamin O." And the promoters still claim that the substance is useful for everything from cancer to arthritis. How do they get around FTC regulations? By adding a disclaimer to the effect that their product

> . . . heals nothing in itself. It helps raise the oxygen level in the bloodstream and cells to the point where the body can naturally keep itself healthier, battle disease and other abnormalities and heal or recover faster. Feeding our bodies more oxygen allows our bodies to more effectively oxidize and metabolize life and health giving nutrients. The information given here is intended for research and educational purposes only and is not intended to prescribe treatment. If you suspect illness you should consult a qualified medical professional.

Of course, they don't address the fact that if their preposterous claims were even remotely true, those people you occasionally encounter toting around oxygen cylinders attached to breathing tubes in their noses would be the healthiest people on earth!

How can anyone continue to make such claims? The FTC simply concedes it lacks the resources to check out every health claim made by advertisers. As with the FDA, it's up to consumers to report advertising fraud and misrepresentation directly to the FTC. Even though the FTC won't resolve individual complaints about ads, if it discerns a pattern of misrepresentations or misleading statements in a dietary supplement's advertisements, it will consider taking action against the company. To file a complaint with the FTC, contact the Consumer Response Center by calling 1-877-FTC-HELP. You can also mail your complaint to Consumer Response Center, Federal Trade Commission, 600 Pennsylvania Avenue NW, Washington, D.C. 20580, or e-mail them using the online complaint form at http://www.ftc.gov/ftc/complaint.htm.

PROTECTING YOUR HEALTH AND YOUR WALLET FROM MEDISCAMMERS

With the incredible number of dietary supplements on the market and the flood of claims associated with them, it's easy to become bewildered. To make matters worse, there's precious little hard scientific evidence to establish the safety and efficacy of such products. Though controlled testing in long-term, well-designed studies is expensive, it's sorely needed in the arena of dietary supplements. At present it's up to the individual consumer to evaluate each supplement based on the limited amount of scientific evidence available. However, there are a number of precautions you can take that will reduce the chances of wasting your money or your health on worthless or inappropriate supplements.

GENERAL CONSIDERATIONS

- The first step in improving your nutritional health is to start eating right. Improve your eating habits so that your diet is well-balanced.

Follow the current dietary guidelines provided by the U.S. government posted at www.health.gov/dietary guidelines.

- Don't self-prescribe if you're having a health problem. Consult a doctor before taking any dietary supplement intended to help remedy an existing problem.
- Check out the claims of any supplement you're considering. Do your homework by doing some independent research. The International Bibliographic Information on Dietary Supplements (IBIDS) is a user-friendly database of published scientific literature on dietary supplements. Produced by ODS at the National Institutes of Health, it can be located on the Internet at http://odp.od.nih.gov/ods/databases/ibids/html. Also check the FDA's Web site to see if there have been any recent warnings or recalls of any supplement you're considering taking.
- Always read carefully the product labels and any information accompanying a supplement. What kinds of claims are included in the product literature? Are the claims and/or clinical proof being asserted for the specific product, or for the type of supplement in general?
- Check the expiration date, since supplements may lose potency over time.
- Follow all directions and don't take any more than the recommended dosage. The more you take, the greater the chances you'll have an adverse reaction to the supplement.
- Consider all the warnings provided. What are the possible side effects? What drug and food interactions could occur?
- Be leery of products sold for considerably less than competing brands. It's possible that the product you end up with *isn't* what it's supposed to be. Cheaper, inferior ingredients may have been used to get the price down.
- Be sure to alert medical personnel and others responsible for your health care about every supplement you take. Ask your doctor about what supplement-drug interactions are possible. And don't forget to provide information about the dosage and concentration that you take.

- Certain individuals shouldn't use supplements without medical supervision; these include the elderly, children, teenagers, chronically ill individuals, pregnant women, or nursing moms.
- If any dietary recommendation seems drastic or extreme to you, get a second opinion from a registered dietitian or a traditional physician who is knowledgeable about nutrition.
- Remember to keep all supplements out of the reach of children. Sixty-four percent of the reports to the American Association of Poison Control Centers in 1998 involved kids younger than six. Many supplement bottles don't have childproof caps. And even though some supplement companies are producing products aimed at children, these supplements lack enough scientific testing to be safe for youngsters.
- When taking a dietary supplement, keep a log of any symptoms or side effects you experience, and talk to your doctor about them.
- Be especially cautious about taking supplements prior to any surgery. It's wise to discuss what you're taking with your surgeon and anesthesiologist several weeks before the surgery takes place.
- As with any type of product, if you experience any adverse side effects, stop taking the supplement and call your doctor.
- To avoid becoming a victim of GHB or other party drugs, don't share a drink with someone else or accept a drink from a punch bowl. To make sure no one slips anything into your drink, never take your eyes off it from the moment it's poured.

GETTING HIGH-QUALITY SUPPLEMENTS

To protect yourself from supplements of inferior quality, the FDA recommends that you:

- Look for ingredients in products with the U.S. Pharmacopeia (USP) notation. This shows that the manufacturer followed standards established by the USP, a not-for-profit group that promotes public health by establishing standards of quality for medicines and other health-care technologies.

- Remember that just because something is "natural" doesn't mean it's safe.
- Look for a nationally known food and drug manufacturer—one that already has manufacturing standards in place for its other products. Although it's no guarantee that the supplement will be of high quality, at the very least the company should have a track record of complying with other tight controls.
- If you have questions, contact the manufacturer directly for information about the conditions under which it manufactures its products.

There is still a lack of information about many supplements, and much of the information furnished by manufacturers is false and misleading despite the efforts of the FDA and FTC to correct such problems. Ultimately the responsibility for choosing appropriate supplements falls squarely on the shoulders of the individual. So be a cautious, skeptical, and well-informed consumer.

chapter 13

Dental MediScams

Taking a Bite Out of Your Wallet

THE DENTIST'S ESTIMATE HAD climbed to $4,748. Six crowns, two fillings and bleaching. That's what he had recommended. But I already knew there was nothing wrong with my teeth.

As if you don't already hate going to the dentist, I'm about to give you a few more reasons to loathe the trip.

Going undercover for a television news show, I visited six different Las Vegas dentists for checkup exams, telling each dentist that my insurance was about to run out.

"Is there any work I need done on my teeth?" I asked.

The first three dentists said my teeth were fine or needed only minimal work. But by the fourth dentist, the estimates started to get expensive.

Dentist #4 suggested I consider getting two teeth capped. "It's totally elective," he said. "Your mouth is in A-1 condition. Those silver fillings could last you a while or they could break. We just never know." The charge for the two caps, charting, and cleaning: $1,317. So far, so good—at least in comparison with what was to come.

My next appointment was with a dentist who had no trouble finding all sorts of problems with my teeth.

"You've got all this erosion down here at the gum line," he told me as I lay in the chair squinting into the blaring lights, my mouth stretched wide open. I could only mumble. "These two here," he continued, "both have decay under the crown on both of those . . . and those crowns should both be replaced." Not only that, he continued, "with those front teeth, at some point, those are going to have to be crowned."

I walked out of Dentist #5's exam with an estimate totaling $3,972. That would have bought me six gold crowns, one filling, evaluation, X rays, and cleaning.

But there was nothing wrong with my teeth! Before the investigation, I had had them checked by Dr. Lawrence J. Warner, dean of the University of Southern California Dental School.

My sixth appointment was with a dentist whose office had just lost electrical power, so he couldn't read my X rays. But that didn't stop him from finding his own variety of issues inside my mouth.

"I think it would be in your best interest to replace that crown," he told me as he prodded at my gums. He went on to explain that "we're kind of taking an approach . . . rather than reactive, kind of a proactive approach trying to prevent a problem."

The price for such "preventive" dentistry? $4,748 for six crowns, two fillings, and bleaching.

Six different dentists, six different estimates—ranging from zero to almost $5,000. And a look at each dentist's chart on my mouth revealed that each dentist had arrived at a different diagnosis.

What if I *weren't* an undercover reporter? What if I *didn't* already know that there was nothing wrong with my teeth? What if I had placed my trust in these dentists? And what if I were an ongoing patient who'd seen the same dentist regularly for many years, as most of us tend to do? Just what are these dentists up to?

John Hunt, general counsel for the Nevada State Board of Dental Examiners, investigates dental-practice complaints and has the power to recommend discipline of errant dentists. I showed him the results of my investigation.

Said Hunt, "It's obvious, when you have such an extreme swing, that somewhere along the line, somebody is out of line. It appears to me there may be individuals who either are greedy, or they don't possess the necessary skill and training to be performing the work."

Which is it—greedy, or incapable? I returned to the dentists with a camera crew, allowing each a chance to defend himself.

The fourth dentist, who'd recommended the capping work totaling $1,317, would not speak with me—at least not without an appointment, said his business manager.

The fifth dentist did not mind offering his side of things. How did he explain his estimate of $3,972 for six gold crowns, one filling, evaluation, X rays, and cleaning? He took the bold route: "You have to be aware of your own body," he explained, standing in the lobby of his office, his arms waving and a half-grin on his face as he looked me in the eye. I nodded along. He continued, "Anybody that goes in and just throws themselves there and says, you know, 'Do what you will,' is a fool." A fool, I thought, who may soon be parted with almost $4,000.

Our highest bidder, the sixth dentist, also took a shot at explaining his estimate totaling almost $5,000. I asked him why his diagnosis didn't match those from any other exam. The young, handsome dentist had a modest, somewhat tinny voice that was far from huffy. "Well, they were probably able to look at your mouth a lot closer than me because as you recall, we were, you know . . . the power was off."

I asked, "So you're saying it could be a misdiagnosis?"

He started a sentence, sputtered, then began anew. "I don't know, you'd have to talk, I think . . . I . . . You know, I wasn't very thorough when I went through because, as I said," he continued, adding a titter, "I didn't have X rays that I felt like were . . . the best."

HOW MANY DENTISTS OVERCHARGE AND OVERTREAT?

These three dentists are not the only ones doing such things, of course; not surprisingly, other undercover investigations of dentists have found similar results. William Ecenbarger, in an article for *Reader's Digest*, visited fifty dentists in twenty-eight states, bringing along his own X ray films and telling the dentists he had ample insurance coverage. Before the reporter began, four dentists verified that he had only one immediate problem: a molar that needed a filling or a crown. Another tooth might cause some disagreement, but even if both teeth were crowned, the total shouldn't have exceeded $1,500.

What did that reporter find? Much the same as I did—that dentists' fees, examinations, and recommendations vary widely. The visits alone cost from $20 to $141. And this was only the beginning: Only twenty-one of the fifty dentists conducted cancer screening as recommended by the American Dental Association, and only fourteen did the recommended periodontal screening. Only twelve of the fifty dentists agreed with the conclusions of the four dentists who performed the initial appraisal, and fifteen failed to find the main problem with the molar. One dentist recommended crowning all the reporter's teeth—at a cost of $13,440. Other estimates ranged from $500 to a whopping $29,850. The reporter also visited a dental school clinic where the student and a department chairman independently suggested capping both teeth, which would have cost $460.

Finally the reporter consulted an advisor with the American Dental Association, asking how consumers can protect themselves from over-treatment and overcharging. The American Dental Association advisor suggested seeking a second or third opinion, especially if there is much work involved. This would at least provide some comfort, the advisor said.

"I got fifty opinions," replied the reporter, "and I am not comforted."

So it would appear that my own Las Vegas investigation was right in line. Left unanswered, however, is another important question: How much would the treatment estimates have run had the dentists been told I had no insurance?

DENTAL QUACKERY

Dental fraud abounds. Although the most common fraudulent activities among dentists are billing for services not rendered and billing for a more expensive procedure than was actually done, dental quackery also exists. The U.S. Senate defines "quackery" as the promotion of unproven medical schemes for profit. That definition doesn't include dentists who are simply incompetent, or those who overcharge or overtreat or misdiagnose their patients. Quack dentists are those who use techniques not approved by the American Dental Association. Probably the most notorious are "psychic dentists" who claim to be able to rid you of your cavities and pull teeth painlessly without using anesthesia. Less infamous are the other dental MediScammers, but their "treatments" are legion. Here's a look at some of the more common scams.

HOLISTIC DENTISTRY

Taking a cue from holistic medicine, some dentists are embracing pseudoscientific theories. These so-called holistic dentists often claim that "optimum" overall health or "wellness" thwarts disease. As such, some holistic dentists make health claims that go far beyond what a dentist should be involved in. Nutrition is often the focus, and patients are directed toward expensive dietary supplements or dental products. Author and dentist John E. Dodes, D.D.S., an expert on dental quackery, has stated that vague terms such as "wellness" are "something for which quacks can get paid when there is nothing wrong with the patient."

Quackbusters Stephen Barrett, M.D., and William T. Jarvis, Ph.D., describe the many problems associated with holistic dentistry on the Quackwatch Web site (www.quackwatch.com). Holistic practitioners may begin with hair analysis, a computerized dietary review, or even a blood-chemistry screening test. What, you might ask, do all these tests that are farmed out to outside laboratories have to do with your teeth?

Very little, it seems. As discussed in chapter 6, hair analysis is useless in gauging your nutritional state. Computer dietary analysis is useful for finding the composition of a person's diet and can be a legitimate tool for dietary counseling. But few dentists are trained or qualified to perform dietary counseling. And what about those blood-chemistry tests? Authentic, though often misinterpreted. Holistic dentists rarely reference the laboratory's standardized range of "normal" results. Instead, they use a much narrower range to define "normality," then tell their patients that anyone whose values fall outside that range is "out of balance." Being "out of balance," naturally, requires treatment; from there, the holistic dentist may suggest overpriced dietary supplements to "balance the body chemistry."

Other problems are real—and the holistic dentists treat those, too. Not surprisingly, they have their own take on things. The bottom line: Patients who allow holistic dentists to treat more than what's in their mouths may suffer in more places than just their purses. A serious illness or condition may go untreated or mistreated. Even worse, some otherwise well patients have developed serious health problems at the hands of holistic dentists.

TMJ DISORDERS

Disorders of the temperomandibular joint (or TMJ—the place where the upper and lower jaws connect) can cause pain and restrict opening of the mouth. A "clicking" when moving the jaw is often a symptom of TMJ disorders, although clicking alone is not considered a problem. Holistic dentists allege that TMJ problems can result in scoliosis (a sideways curvature of the spine), premenstrual syndrome, and sexual problems—claims not supported by scientific evidence. In fact, studies show that 80 to 90 percent of patients with TMJ pain get better within three months if treated with nonprescription analgesics, moist heat, and exercises—you know, simple, inexpensive stuff. But TMJ has been a hot area for dentists, and the solutions offered by MediScammers are rarely simple and almost never inexpensive.

A Louisiana woman began experiencing popping and clicking in her jaw, along with pain in her ears following the removal of her tonsils and adenoids in 1987. A friend referred her to a dentist who specialized in treating TMJ disorders. The friend might just as well have referred her to a torture chamber.

The dentist recommended a two-phase treatment. In the first phase, the patient was fitted with an "anterior repositioning device" known as the Gelb appliance, which is basically a splint designed to push the lower jaw forward. The patient had to wear the Gelb appliance twenty-four hours a day, returning often to the dentist for tweaking. All the while, she was in constant pain, could only eat soft foods, had trouble walking, and had problems sleeping. She lost almost twenty pounds.

Two months later, still in pain, she saw an orthodontist who recommended that she stop using the Gelb appliance immediately. She didn't listen, and instead returned to the dentist who had installed the device.

In the next phase of her treatment, the quack dentist removed the Gelb appliance and fitted her with another device, an "upper-palate expander." Her pain surged, and her palate became swollen and sensitive.

Finally the woman had the device removed, and discontinued treatment ten months after it had begun. In May 1991 she sought out the orthodontist who had fitted her with braces when she was an adolescent. He discovered that the upper-palate expander had pushed her teeth out beyond her jaw, exposing the roots of her upper molars. Ouch!

The woman sued the so-called TMJ specialist for malpractice, and in 1998 a trial court awarded her $72,800 in damages. An appellate court added another $3,000 for future dental care—to cover the "definite future need for realignment of her lower teeth."

Some practitioners treat TMJ by correcting a patient's "bad bite" (when the teeth do not align correctly with each other). Certain treatments are irreversible, such as grinding down teeth or building them up with dental restorations. Drs. Barrett and Jarvis warn that one commonly used treatment for a bad bite—which involves the placement of a mandibular orthopedic repositioning appliance (MORA) between the teeth—is unproven. These plastic appliances usually cover just some of the teeth and are worn continuously for months or even years. And they do reposition—when worn too much, MORAs can push teeth so far out of proper alignment that orthodontics or facial-reconstructive surgery are necessary to correct the resulting deformity.

"CRANIAL OSTEOPATHY" AND RELATED SCAMS

Proponents of "cranial osteopathy," "craniosacral therapy," "cranial therapy," and similar treatments claim that the skull bones can be manipulated to relieve pain (especially TMJ pain) as well as to correct many other ailments. Although proponents frequently include physical therapists, osteopaths, and chiropractors, some dentists also adhere to this theory.

According to the theory behind these treatments, a rhythm exists in the flow of the cerebrospinal fluid that surrounds the brain and spinal cord. Thus, diseases can be diagnosed by detecting aberrations in this rhythm, then corrected by manipulating the skull.

This theory is not only false, but downright illogical. The bones of the skull are fused to each other in adults and cannot be moved. The idea that you can "manipulate" these bones to affect the underlying cerebrospinal fluid is akin to saying that you can alter the contents of a hen's egg by manipulating the shell. Further, the cerebrospinal fluid does not have a detectable "rhythm." In a recent test, three physical therapists examined the same twelve patients for the "skull-fluid rhythm." All diagnosed significantly different rhythms.

AURICULOTHERAPY

A popular course of study among holistic dentists is auriculotherapy, a form of acupuncture based on the belief that the body and organs are connected to various points on the ear's surface. Dentists insert and twirl needles or administer small electrical currents at points on the ear to relieve facial pains or treat other trouble spots in the body. Negative side effects include complications from unsterile and broken needles.

BAD-BREATH TREATMENTS

Dr. Stephen Barrett states that another problem area for consumers is a topic many don't like to discuss. Although some dentists claim to specialize in the treatment of bad breath, they have no special expertise in the area. Apparently they're primarily interested in increasing their income by selling unproven products. Through multilevel marketing, the makers of one such product offer unsubstantiated claims that their product eliminates mouth odors, cleans teeth, and conditions gums (whatever "conditions" may mean). According to Barrett, the active ingredient is chlorine dioxide, which is also used as an algaecide in swimming pools.

Enough said.

CAVITATIONAL OSTEOPATHOSIS

Even though there's no scientific proof to support their theories, proponents of this form of dubious dentistry maintain that facial pain, heart disease, arthritis, and other health problems can be caused by infected "cavitations" within the jaw bones that are not detectable by X ray or treatable with antibiotics. The condition—"cavitational osteopathosis" or "neuralgia-inducing cavitational osteonecrosis"—can only be cured by locating and scraping out the affected tissues. Believers may also remove all root-canal–treated teeth and most of the vital teeth close to the infected area. Needless to say, the lack of legitimate scientific proof has never stopped a good MediScammer from charging an arm and a leg for bogus treatments that do the patient much harm and no good whatever.

All things considered, I think I'd prefer the Gelb appliance.

MERCURY-AMALGAM TOXICITY

Not to be outdone, some dentists still claim the mercury in silver-mercury amalgam fillings is toxic. You know the story by now: Toxic mercury from your fillings leaks into your system and leads to a wide range of health problems, including MS, arthritis, headaches, Parkinson's disease, emotional stress, and so on and on. And you thought the original cavities themselves were bad!

Without even searching for references to amalgams, I found one Web site on prostate-cancer therapies which discussed the controversial subject of amalgam toxicity. While cautioning the reader to do his own research, the author, a prostate-cancer survivor, concludes that the evidence in support of amalgam toxicity is overwhelming because of the number of patients who have experienced dramatic improvement after mercury is removed from their mouths and bodies. According to his Web site, cleansing of the mouth controls the body energetically and physically. He goes on to describe the mixture of metals commonly contained in the mouth as a type of "battery in the mouth." He states that the most common mouth metal is the dental amalgam, which is 50 percent mercury, a very toxic substance. While the government makes it a felony to put one drop of mercury in the ground, he continues, the government and even mainstream dentistry still endorse the amalgam in the mouth.

The "toxic mercury" fighters recommend your silver fillings be replaced with either gold or plastic ones; some go even further and tell you to take vitamin supplements to prevent trouble during the process. Never mind that scientific testing has shown again and again that the amount of mercury absorbed from fillings is negligible. According to the American Dental Association, "People are exposed to more total mercury from food, water, and air than from the minuscule amounts of mercury vapor generated from amalgam fillings." Keep in mind here that if the dental profession had even a shred of reliable evidence that amalgam fillings really were toxic, every dentist in the country would be making a fortune removing mercury fillings and replacing them with gold or plastic fillings. But the American Dental Association, as the organization that speaks for ethical dentistry, recognizes that amalgam fillings have an indisputable safety record.

Nor does the American Dental Association stand alone on this position. The U.S. Public Health Service issued a report in 1993 stating there is no valid health-related reason for not using silver-mercury fillings except in the extremely rare case of the patient who is allergic to a component of amalgam. This conclusion is supported by the independent findings of the FDA, the National Institutes of Health Technology Assessment Conference, and the National Institutes of Dental Research. In

1991 *Consumer Reports* noted that mercury-amalgam fillings are still the consumer's best bet.

The U.S. Public Health Service found it inadvisable to remove amalgam fillings due to the structural damage that could occur to healthy teeth. Furthermore, the American Dental Association Council on Ethics, Bylaws, and Judicial Affairs considers the unnecessary removal of silver-amalgam fillings "improper and unethical."

End of story? Hardly.

Enter the Dental Potentiometer. This device, which is nothing more than a simple electric meter like you'd buy at a retail electronics store, displays a number when its probe is applied to a surface— any surface. Unethical dentists have used this meter to persuade patients to have their amalgam fillings replaced. The dentists claimed the numeric reading represented the electrical activity of mercury leaching into the body. Based on "data" supplied by the probe, patients could decide which of their fillings needed replacing first.

One of the most strident advocates of amalgam toxicity has been Hal A. Huggins, D.D.S., a former dentist who practiced in Colorado Springs, Colorado. As far back as 1975 the American Dental Association Council on Dental Research had denounced a special diet Huggins had been promoting. But that didn't deter Huggins. In the mid-1980s, the FDA forced Huggins to stop marketing mineral products he claimed would aid in ridding the body of mercury. Huggins also believed that root-canal therapy could make people susceptible to arthritis, MS, ALS, and other autoimmune diseases, despite the lack of objective evidence to support such theories.

On the other hand, Huggins' "treatments" could be distinctly detrimental to your health. Take the case of one young woman who was thirty-six in 1991 when she watched a broadcast of CBS's *60 Minutes* that featured Huggins and his "theories." After viewing other tapes and reading portions of Huggins' book, *It's All in Your Head: Diseases Caused by Mercury Amalgam Fillings,* she made an appointment at Huggins' clinic. She was immediately struck by the beauty of the facility, as well as the positive attitude of Huggin's associate, the dentist who took care of her. Convinced by these superficial trappings of legitimacy, the young woman—who did not have dental problems when she entered the clinic—allowed Huggins' associate to remove and replace nine amalgam fillings, as well as extract three teeth that had undergone root-canal treatment. The woman soon developed nagging facial pains. She ultimately sued Huggins for malpractice, and in 1996 won a $159,000 award against him and his clinic.

That same year, Huggins' dental license was finally revoked. The administrative-law judge who presided over the revocation proceedings concluded that Huggins had diagnosed mercury toxicity in every patient seen in his clinic, *even in patients who didn't have mercury fillings*. Huggins also had recommended to his patients that any teeth that had undergone root-canal therapy should be pulled. The judge concluded that Huggins' treatments were "a sham, illusory and without scientific basis."

In comparison to those who visited Huggins, I seem to have gotten off lucky in my own investigation!

BEWARE OF DENTAL "PIONEERS"

According to Dr. Dodes, Americans spend well over a billion dollars a year on quack dentistry—and that's just for medically unproven treatments. If you add in insurance fraud and the costs of misdiagnosis and overtreatment, the costs are far higher.

Dentists are trained to take care of your teeth and mouth. They are not trained in general medicine, chiropractic, or nutrition. So beware of the dentist who tries to act like a physician, chiropractor, or nutritionist; and be especially wary of "pioneering" dentists like Huggins who try to convince you that everything your previous dentists have done for you—not to mention the entire dental profession itself—has been wrong. More often than not, the "maverick" dentist is a MediScammer pure and simple, who will charge you outrageous sums of money for treatments that, at best, you don't need. Of course, as we've seen, even "mainstream" dentists can overcharge and overtreat. But at least their main threat is not to your health but to your wallet—or the coffers of your insurance company.

Well, did I give you a few more reasons to hate to go to the dentist? If so, *don't* be deterred from going to a reputable one. The overall advantages of good dental health and regular trips to the dentist far and above outweigh the risks. And you can tip the scales even further in your favor by being a smart consumer of dental services. Here's how:

- Check out the dentist before you become a patient. Call the board of dental examiners in your state capital and ask if the dentist has been the subject of any disciplinary actions.
- Don't be afraid to ask for second or third opinions. Even competent, ethical dentists sometimes disagree. Especially if you're facing high-dollar procedures, make sure the money really needs to be spent.
- If the dentist promises to "cure" a disease unrelated to your teeth or mouth, *run*. Likewise avoid a dentist who tries to sell you nutritional supplements or other goods or services unrelated to dentistry.
- If the dentist offers you a treatment or procedure you've never heard of, check it out with the American Dental Association (see appendix) before you submit to it. If they've never heard of it, or specifically disapprove of it, there's an excellent chance the dentist offering it is a MediScammer.
- Always check your bills. When you visit a dentist, understand what fees your insurance should cover and what fees you are responsible for yourself.

chapter 14

Spotting the MediScams

The Telltale Tip-offs and
Profiles of Medical Quacks and Their Victims

JASON (NOT HIS REAL NAME), thirty-four, had lung cancer. After continual trips to his doctors and repeated failures with conventional medicine, he had almost given up hope—until he heard about a Southern California clinic with an innovative alternative treatment. Disgusted that his doctors and modern medicine had been unable to cure him, Jason and his wife, Martha (not her real name), decided to investigate.

Jason and Martha met Lawrence Taylor, a licensed general practitioner and "co-discoverer," along with his chemist partner, William Stacey, of Immunostim. The procedure was simple: The substance would be administered by IV into one of Jason's veins for three to six hours, four times a week, for three weeks.

The first treatment, though painful, was without incident. During the second treatment, however, the solution leaked onto Jason's hand. He immediately felt excruciating, burning pain that intensified over the next few hours. Even though the nurse administered large doses of pain medication, it brought little relief. The couple continued the treatments at home, still hoping that Jason would be cured.

Several months later, following an in-home Immunostim treatment, Jason was left in such pain that he had to be rushed to the hospital. The doctors there gave him the narcotic pain reliever Demerol, which he continued to take after leaving the hospital. However, he had lost the use of his hand below the IV injection site and did not regain its use until a week later. The Immunostim treatments had cost the couple nearly $26,000 and had done absolutely nothing to slow the progress of Jason's cancer, let alone cure it. And because the couple had squandered most of their assets on these worthless treatments, Martha was left with serious financial problems.

The clinic run by Taylor and his partner administered Immunostim to patients from all over the U.S. who'd heard about this "miracle drug" by word of mouth. These patients paid up to $7,500 per treatment to have Immunostim injected into their veins. Altogether, Taylor and Stacey took in more than $670,000 in eighteen months.

During the subsequent FDA investigation, a review of the clinic's medical records showed that most of the patients who were treated experienced painful inflammation of the veins in which the substance was administered. One witness talked about a patient who writhed in pain on the floor because "he was in too much pain to sit."

An analysis of the Immunostim solution by the FDA's Forensic Chemistry Center identified it as consisting mostly of water and caustic alkaline chemicals, the type found in automatic dish detergents, disinfectants, and toilet-bowl cleaners. No active drug ingredients were present, and the solution had a dangerously high pH of 12.7, compared with a normal blood pH of about 7.4. This almost certainly accounted for the painful reactions of many patients.

Although Taylor was a real physician, Stacey, who claimed to have a Ph.D. in chemistry, probably had no more than a high school education. In May 1995 both men pleaded no contest to criminal fraud charges in a plea bargain. Taylor was sentenced to a 150-day work-furlough facility and three years' probation, was fined $2,000, and had to pay for the cost of the investigation. His medical license was later revoked, and he and Stacey also had to pay restitution of $46,779 to 9 of the 108 former patients or their families. By the time of sentencing, more than half of the clinic's patients had died, presumably from their diseases. Stacey was sentenced to eighteen months in jail with five years' probation, ordered to pay $3,000 in fines, and ordered not to sell health care products or even to work in the industry again. Stacey failed to appear to begin his jail sentence and eventually was found in South Carolina, still selling Immunostim. He was sentenced to five years in prison, the maximum penalty allowed under the plea-bargain agreement.

TELLTALE TIP-OFFS

Could Jason and Martha have avoided this MediScam? Were there adequate warnings to indicate to them that something just wasn't right about Dr. Taylor's clinic? Absolutely. Here's just a partial list of the tip-offs that should have alerted the couple to the fact that they were about to get scammed.

- **The treatment was available nowhere else.** This is the number one tip-off that something is wrong. If a drug is approved by the FDA, any doctor is permitted to prescribe it. Even if the drug is considered "experimental," and therefore not yet FDA-approved, there will be multiple sites where you can obtain such treatment. Before shelling out money for a treatment you've never heard of, do some research. Contact the Centers for Disease Control and Prevention in Atlanta or a relevant support group like the American Heart Association or the American Cancer Society for information about the treatment (I've included a list of such organizations, along with phone numbers and Web sites in the appendix). If they haven't heard of the treatment, it's a sure bet that it's bogus. Above all, don't fall for the standard quack's line that his or her research is being "suppressed" by the mainstream medical community for reasons of professional jealousy. If a cure—any cure—is legitimate, the medical and scientific communities will rush to embrace it. Anyone who tells you different is either naïve, paranoid, or a liar.

- **The physician was not a specialist in the diseases he was treating.** While general practitioners, general internists, and family physicians certainly have a distinguished place in providing medical care, one obviously would expect a cancer specialist called an oncologist, to know more about cancer than a non-specialist. Yet Taylor, a general practitioner, claimed to have secrets to curing cancer that no oncologist was aware of. A quick call to the county or state medical association, the state board of medical examiners, or the specific specialty board is all it takes to determine what diseases a particular physician is specialized to treat. If a non-specialist offers treatments you can't get from a specialist, watch out!

- **The clinic used mostly testimonials to tout its treatment.** As we saw in chapter 10, the placebo effect is a very powerful force. One-third or more of patients receiving a placebo or sham treatment will report noticeable improvement—that makes it easy for any doctor to gather patient testimonials for even a totally bogus treatment. Physicians offering legitimate therapies usually refer to published statistics when discussing success rates, as in "three out of four patients who undergo this therapy are cancer-free five years later." And be wary of the physician who claims success rates approaching 100 percent. Ask where those numbers come from, and be skeptical if they're not published in a reputable medical journal you can look up yourself. Universal success is rare in medicine.

- **The physician promised a "cure."** Physicians rarely "promise" a good outcome, let alone a cure. In the first place, such promises are considered a contract of sorts, and leave the physician open to a lawsuit if results fall short of such promises—even if the physician carried out the treatment flawlessly. More importantly, an ethical physician doesn't want to build up false hopes. Quacks, on the other hand, know that patients desperately want to hear words like "cure" and will more readily shell out the bucks when they do. Always beware the physician who promises you exactly what you want to hear, especially if you've already been told that your condition is incurable.

BOGUS DOCTORS—
Just How Easy Is It to Fake a Medical Degree?

When we seek medical care, we naturally assume that the doctor who examines and treats us is a legitimate medical school graduate. Yet every year we read reports about "doctors" caught practicing without a license or practicing after their licenses have been revoked. Think about it. Do you know for a fact that every doctor you've ever seen had proper credentials?

Stolen Identities

The success of bogus doctors in carrying out their charades varies enormously. Some are so inept they give themselves away within a matter of weeks or months. But others, those with a high IQ or a photographic memory along with a health-related background, have gone undetected for years. And of these, the most successful are usually those who cover their tracks—at least partially—by assuming the identity of a legitimate physician.

Take the strange case of Gerald Barnbaum. Trained as a pharmacist, Barnbaum prided himself on his medical knowledge and ability to diagnose diseases from symptoms alone. In 1976, after losing his Illinois pharmacy license as the result of a Medicaid fraud investigation, Barnbaum decided to put his other skills to work. He moved to California where he pulled the name of a real California doctor with a name similar to his own out of a medical directory. He legally adopted the same name, then had letterheads printed. With this stationery he wrote to the California Board of Medicine requesting copies of "his" medical license, saying the original had been burned in a fire. Barnbaum then used the license to receive copies of the real doctor's diplomas and other records.

With these credentials in hand, Barnbaum got a job as a physician with a Los Angeles clinic. After a year without apparent incident, he switched to a higher-paying position in Orange County. Then, in 1979, Barnbaum examined a twenty-nine-year-old man who complained he had lost a lot of weight, and was dizzy and constantly thirsty. Although these are classic symptoms of rapid-onset diabetes, Barnbaum ordered some tests and then gave the patient a tranquilizer and sent him home. Two days later the man was found dead of advanced diabetes.

Barnbaum's charade was discovered in the subsequent investigation, and he was charged with practicing medicine without a license and involuntary manslaughter. Out on bail awaiting trial, Barnbaum was again hired as a physician by a Los Angeles clinic. This time he was arrested on his first day at the new job.

Barnbaum pleaded guilty to the charges against him and spent the next three years in prison. He used this time to study medicine in the library and through correspondence courses. Out on parole in 1983, he worked in sales until his parole ended the next year. Then he took his collection of medical credentials and found work as a doctor at a series of clinics, none of which bothered to verify his background. A hospital affiliated with one of the clinics did check up on him, though, and discovered the ruse. After three months of practicing medicine, Barnbaum was again arrested and sentenced to another three years in prison.

After serving his sentence, Barnbaum was arrested and reimprisoned in 1989 and 1991, again on charges related to impersonation of a physician. He was released in 1992 and, yet again, resumed his charade. He apparently hopped from one clinic to the next, quickly moving on whenever suspicions about his credentials were raised. Finally, in 1996, he was caught again and pleaded guilty to charges including mail fraud and illegal prescribing. He was sentenced to another three years in prison.

Is Barnbaum's charade over? In 1996, while in jail awaiting trial, Barnbaum wrote to the alma mater of the doctor whose identity he'd stolen requesting a copy of "his" medical diploma. This time, however, the school declined his request.

Another example of a bogus doctor who succeeded by stealing a real physician's identity was "Dr. J. D. Phillips," who practiced medicine for thirty years. He was said to have fooled patients in eleven states, the U.S. government, county and state health departments, as well as physicians, administrators, and nurses. He was eventually sentenced to fifteen to twenty years in prison for perjury.

Bogus doctors are often so attentive and compassionate with their patients that they continue to enjoy a loyal following even after they are exposed. Take the case of one Freddie Brant, an ex-con who launched his medical career in a prison hospital. Later, he assumed the identity of a doctor he had worked for in Tennessee. Using the doctor's medical license, Brant obtained a reciprocal license in Texas without having to take any examinations. He then became a staff doctor at the State Hospital in Texas. He later moved on to the small village of Groveton, Texas, where he became the town physician. He was exposed when he and the real doctor, who was still in Tennessee, happened to order drugs on the same day from the same pharmaceutical firm.

The citizens of Groveton supported Brant even when he was charged with forgery and impersonating a doctor; the grand jury refused to indict him. His perjury trial ended with a hung jury. Why did those he deceived remain so loyal to him? For one thing, he was a willing listener who inspired confidence in his patients. For another, he made house calls and charged only $5 for the service and $3 for office visits. And few patients appear to have been harmed by his lack of formal medical education, especially since he referred difficult cases to legitimate doctors. There have been other cases in which the former patients have gone so far as to circulate petitions to prevent the bogus doctors from being prosecuted.

A Charismatic Impostor

Not all bogus doctors go to the trouble of stealing a real doctor's identity. Sometimes all the impostor needs is confidence and charisma. Take the case of Frank Abagnale, who posed as an airline pilot, a doctor, an attorney, and a college professor—all between the ages of sixteen and twenty-one!

On the run from the F.B.I. as a result of his confidence games, Abagnale hadn't originally planned to work as a doctor. He only listed himself as "Dr. Frank Williams," a non-practicing physician from Los Angeles, when he rented an apartment in a singles complex in Atlanta. Soon everyone around him was calling him "Doc" and asking for medical advice. Abagnale generally told them to see their own doctors.

A couple of months later, Abagnale's new neighbor knocked on his door and introduced himself as the chief resident pediatrician for a local hospital. Instead of moving somewhere else, Abagnale decided to avoid him. But the neighbor was lonely and often stopped Abagnale on his way to his car, the swimming pool, tennis court, and so on. So Abagnale visited Emory University's medical library every day to read journals on pediatric medicine. Then, when the doctor came home after a long day, Abagnale would wait for him and discuss what he'd read that day.

One afternoon the doctor invited Abagnale to visit a new hospital that was just opening. After Abagnale's visit, everyone he'd met—doctors, nurses, administrators, and orderlies alike—was convinced he was a pediatrician from Los Angeles. Abagnale began dating a nurse who worked at the hospital, and he could often be found waiting for her in the lobby.

Eventually an administrator for the hospital offered Abagnale a job filling in on the midnight-to-eight shift for an intern who needed to take an emergency leave. When Abagnale replied that he didn't have a license to practice medicine in Georgia, the administrator said he could get a verbal okay from the medical-review board and have him start the next night.

Unwilling to pass up a challenge, Abagnale accepted and—at the age of eighteen—found himself working as a doctor in a hospital. It didn't matter that he knew nothing about the hospital procedures, or that he hated the sight of blood. He simply avoided medical duties by burying himself in administrative tasks. At times he was called down to the emergency room when an intern had a question. Abagnale rarely saw a patient, but instead would aggressively walk in and order the intern to follow standard procedure, then walk out again. The interns liked him for this.

Abagnale wound up working an entire year at the hospital before a replacement for him was found. He then resigned and left on his own, with no one the wiser. During that year he never diagnosed a patient or administered drugs, but acted solely as an administrator. And he had a good excuse for avoiding patient-care duties—under Georgia law, his temporary license did not allow him to administer drugs or to examine, diagnose, or treat patients.

A harmless prank? Hardly. Even Abagnale later admitted that it bothered him that his illegible, meaningless scribblings in the patients' charts *never* had been questioned by the hospital staff.

While some impostors may use the excuse that they never harmed a patient, how do they really know that? Consider the time that the victim wasted seeing an impostor when diagnoses and treatments by a real doctor could have been provided. Often, early detection of a disease is critical to a cure.

NOT ALL "DOCTORS" ARE REALLY M.D.'S

Fewer cases of "successful" impersonation of medical doctors have been revealed in recent years due to stricter licensing procedures. But what if the doctor *doesn't pretend* to be an M.D. and the patient doesn't know the difference? That kind of confusion caused one woman to get much of her face burned away by skin creams given her by the wrong kind of doctor.

She originally went to a popular doctor, who had been recommended by some acquaintances, when she experienced arthritis pains in her shoulder. She received "chiropractic-type treatment" and acupuncture which relieved some of the pain. When she mentioned a sore on her nose, the doctor said it could be skin cancer and sold her a $10 jar of his "black salve" to be administered three times a day. The salve caused painful red burns around the sore and on her cheeks. The doctor told her the redness proved the sore was cancerous, and directed her to put the salve on the red areas. The burns worsened and, on her return visit, the doctor sold her "white salve" to relieve the pain.

The woman's condition deteriorated and, after waiting five days, she got a second opinion. The doctors at the local hospital told her the salve was "more caustic than oven cleaner" and by then most of the skin on her nose, cheeks, and upper lip had been burned away.

An investigation into the doctor's background revealed that he was not a medical doctor but a naturopath. A naturopath treats patients with herbal remedies, homeopathy, massage, heat, and similar therapies. Although naturopaths may use the title "doctor" and refer to themselves as "physicians," they are not allowed to prescribe drugs or conduct surgery or other invasive procedures. In most states they are not licensed or even regulated. They use the letters "N.D." instead of "M.D." after their names, making it easy for some patients to confuse them with medical doctors. Because the naturopath who treated the woman did not hold himself out to be an M.D., it was difficult for the authorities to crack down on him.

The woman sued for damages, but the naturopath declared bankruptcy to avoid financial liability. As far as I know, the naturopath is still practicing his trade.

Again, a quick call to the state medical board to verify the doctor's credentials would have saved this patient much pain and grief.

ENTER THE INTERNET

One of the more frightening aspects of the Internet is that it has created a gigantic opportunity for quacks and bogus doctors. Not only can they now reach millions of people with their scams, but they can do it from outside the U.S. borders, making them nearly immune from prosecution. Already, prescription drugs like Viagra and Xanax are readily available over the Internet. All the patient has to do is answer a few quick questions and provide a credit card number and the prescription will be on its way. Sometimes the patient gets the real drugs, sometimes a look-alike counterfeit. Sometimes a real doctor is behind the operation, sometimes a quack. In either case, organized medicine takes a dim view of such practices. In March 2000, Steven Moos, a general practitioner from suburban Portland, Oregon, was fined $5,000 and placed on ten years' probation for prescribing drugs over the Internet. The penalties were levied by the Oregon Board of Medical Examiners, who called the practice "unprofessional and dishonorable." Moos was one of at least twelve doctors nationwide to be censured for prescribing over the Internet.

In *FDA Consumer*, Carol Lewis recounts the tale of Edwin E. Kokes, a quack who posed as a doctor over the Internet. He claimed that he could diagnose AIDS, cancer, allergies, and a host of other problems from hair and fingernail samples. Not only that, but he claimed he could cure those same diseases. Some of those who responded to his Internet solicitations were referred to his office; others were diagnosed and treated through the mails.

Kokes charged between $25 and $50 for each sample he analyzed, then prescribed drugs not approved by the FDA. One "drug" cost $300 for a four-ounce bottle. The FDA's analysis of the product found that it was nothing more than diluted sulfuric acid. Not surprisingly, a patient had complained that the product had burned her skin when she applied it topically.

During the subsequent FDA investigation, an undercover case agent was told by Kokes that he had cured four hundred to five hundred AIDS patients and 97 percent of his three to four thousand ovarian-cancer patients. He said he advised his patients not to seek out traditional treatment as that could worsen the condition or cause death. Some of his patients were even made to sign a waiver agreeing to keep their office visits confidential. The FDA found that he had generated almost $1 million in seven years.

Kokes was charged with eleven counts of mail fraud and one count of practicing under a fictitious name or title. All but one count of mail fraud was dropped in a plea-bargain agreement in which he received the maximum penalty allowed for the charge that stuck. He was fined $5,000, ordered to pay $80,000 in restitution to his victims, and was sentenced to two-and-a-half years in prison and three years of supervised release.

The Internet truly is the new frontier for quackery and MediScams. Almost anyone can now pretend to be a doctor and offer bogus diagnoses and treatments, especially if done from an offshore base. But keep this in mind: No competent, ethical physician would even consider offering a diagnosis or treatment without first examining and interviewing the patient *in person*. You can get many things over the Internet these days; quality health care is not one of them.

AVOIDING THE QUACKS

Even intelligent, educated, and otherwise sensible people are sometimes taken in by quacks. That's especially true when they're driven by fear and desperation because conventional medicine has failed them. But squandering money on a quack cure accomplishes nothing at best, and at worst wastes valuable time and resources. So before you fall for a MediScam, consider the following.

- Don't spend your money before you've done your research. Check out your doctor's credentials with the state medical board and the local medical society before you go. Be aware that impostors sometimes steal the identities of real doctors.
- Be *extremely* suspicious of anyone who claims to be able to cure an incurable disease. Keep in mind the tried and true saying: if it sounds to good to be true, it probably is.
- Don't be fooled by medical jargon. Just because you as a layman can't understand what someone is saying doesn't mean it makes good medical sense. It's easy to start with an accepted, scientifically proven statement and end up with mumbo jumbo.
- Don't accept testimonials as proof that a treatment or cure is effective. Remember that, because of the placebo effect, even blatantly fraudulent treatments produce legions of "satisfied patients." Also remember that if the only support for the product is provided through personal success stories, without statistics or published scientific literature to back them up, the product is most likely bogus.
- Be suspicious of anyone who claims to be the only source of the treatment. As Ben Wilson, M.D., a long-time member of the NCRHI told me, "No real pioneer keeps his results to himself."

- Beware of money-back guarantees. It's unlikely you'll ever receive a refund. The high cost of a treatment alone may be a red flag.
- Head for the exit if someone maintains that he or she is being persecuted by the medical establishment. This claim is the hallmark of a MediScammer.
- Be suspicious if your doctor makes you sign a confidentiality agreement or becomes angry if you request a second opinion. Both of these are unethical practices.
- Be cautious if a health clinic requires you to travel and stay far from your home for treatment. Check out the clinic and its physicians through the state's medical board before you go. Be especially dubious of foreign clinics.
- Report suspected quacks to your state medical board.

Final Thoughts

As I said in the introduction, my purpose in writing this book was not to disparage those in the medical profession. Most doctors are kind, dedicated, and competent professionals who are worthy of our trust. Yet the medical community doesn't do nearly enough to weed out the incompetent, impaired, and downright bogus doctors. And while various government agencies try to crack down on the con artists and other MediScammers offering fraudulent medical products and services, the fact is that these operations crop up far faster than the agencies can react against them. Further, many well-intentioned people are out there offering bogus medical products they honestly believe are beneficial. That's why it's important for each of us to be aware of what's going on, to do our own research into our treatment options, and to check out the credentials of our doctor or other caregiver before we entrust our health and perhaps even our very lives to that person.

This book has not attempted to be a thorough compendium of every MediScam out there. Rather, I've tried to provide you with a broad overview of the breadth and pervasiveness of the schemes being carried out by those who would pocket your health care dollars under false pretenses. Instead of listing every questionable product and treatment—and new ones pop up every day—in MediScams, I've tried to raise your level of awareness of just how easy it is to be taken in by them. Most important, I've tried to point out the common threads and telltale signs that will help you identify a MediScam in action, and provide some common-sense tips for making sure that the health care you receive—and pay for—is both legitimate and necessary.

In conclusion, I hope that the stories, information, and views I've presented in this book will make you a little more thoughtful and a lot more cautious before you dole out money for what you assume is good health care but just might be a MediScam.

Appendix: Resources

ABC

www.abcnews.go.com/sections/living

News and information about health-related issues.

Administration on Aging (AoA)

330 Independence Avenue SW

Washington, D.C. 20201

1-202-619-7501 (National Aging Info Center for technical info and public inquiries.)

1-800-677-1116 (Monday to Friday, 9 A.M. to 8 P.M. Eastern time) (Eldercare Locator; ask for the local ombudsman program or area agency on aging in your area.)

e-mail: aoainfo@aoa.gov

www.aoa.gov

Has information about choosing a nursing home and fact sheets on health issues for seniors.

American Academy of Medical Acupuncture (AAMA)

5820 Wilshire Boulevard, Suite 500

Los Angeles, CA 90036

1-800-521-2262

1-323-937-5514

www.medicalacupuncture.org

Provides information about acupuncture. Call to find a credentialed (physician) provider.

American Association of Retired Persons (AARP)

601 E Street NW

Washington, D.C. 20049

1-800-424-3410

1-202-434-2277

e-mail: member@aarp.org

www.aarp.org

Membership organization of persons fifty years of age or older, working or retired. AARP seeks to promote quality of life for older people. Provides information on health issues, how to choose a nursing home, and fraud.

American Board of Medical Specialties (ABMS)

1007 Church Street, Suite 404

Evanston, IL 60201-5913

1-847-491-9091 *or* 1-866-ASK-ABMS (Call between 9 A.M. and 6 P.M. Eastern time.)

fax: 1-847-328-3596

www.abms.org *or* www.certifieddoctor.org

This organization certifies specialty boards. Call to see if a physician's certifying board is ABMS-approved. The Certified Doctor Verification Service contains the names of the members certified by an ABMS member board.

American Board of Plastic Surgery (ABPS)

Seven Penn Center, Suite 400

1635 Market Street

Philadelphia, PA 19103-2204

1-215-587-9322

fax: 1-215-587-9622

www.abplsurg.org

Certifies plastic surgeons.

American Botanical Council (ABC)

P.O. Box 144345

Austin, TX 78714-4345

1-512-926-4900

fax: 1-512-926-2345

www.herbalgram.org

ABC's goals are to educate the public about beneficial herbs and plants and to promote the safe and effective use of medicinal plants.

American Cancer Society

1-800-ACS-2345

www.cancer.org

Has information about cancer and its treatment.

American Chiropractic Association

1701 Clarendon Boulevard

Arlington, VA 22209

1-800-986-4636

fax: 1-703-243-2593

www.amerchiro.org

Call to find a credentialed provider.

American College of Physicians–American Society of Internal Medicine (ACP–ASIM)

Annals of Internal Medicine

Headquarters: 190 North Independence Mall West

Philadelphia, PA 19106-1572

1-800-523-1546 ext. 2600 *or* 1-215-351-2600

www.acponline.org

Has information on internal medicine and fraud.

American Council on Science and Health (ACSH)

1995 Broadway, 2nd Floor

New York, NY 10023-5860

1-212-362-7044

fax: 1-212-362-4919

www.acsh.org

Nonprofit consumer education agency providing the public with mainstream scientific information on issues such as food, nutrition, pharmaceuticals, the environment, and health.

American Dental Association

211 East Chicago Avenue

Chicago, IL 60611

1-312-440-2500

fax: 1-312-440-2800

www.ada.org

Offers information on dentistry and membership directory. Publishes *Journal of the American Dental Association (JADA)*.

American Diabetes Association

National Office

1701 North Beauregard Street

Alexandria, VA 22311

1-800-DIABETES *or* 1-800-342-2383

e-mail: customerservice@diabetes.org

www.diabetes.org

Contact for information about diabetes and its treatment.

American Dietetic Association

216 West Jackson Boulevard

Chicago, IL 60606-6995

1-312-899-0040 *or* 1-800-366-1655

1-900-225-5267 (to talk to a registered dietician)

www.eatright.org

Offers a consumer hotline where your questions about nutritional supplements can be answered. Call to find a registered dietician.

American Heart Association
National Center
7272 Greenville Avenue
Dallas, TX 75231
Customer Heart and Stroke Information: 1-800-AHA-USA1
www.amhrt.org *or* www.americanheart.org
Gives information on heart disease.

American Medical Association (AMA)
Headquarters: 515 North State Street
Chicago, IL 60610
1-312-464-5000
www.ama-assn.org
National professional association of physicians that sets standards for the medical profession. Has information on HIV, AIDS, asthma, migraine, women's health, etc. Publishes the *Journal of the American Medical Association (JAMA)*.

American Society of Aesthetic Plastic Surgery (ASAPS)
Cosmetic Plastic Surgery Referral Line: 1-888-272-7711
www.surgery.org
Call to obtain a list of ASAPS members in your area.

American Society of Plastic Surgeons (ASPS)
444 East Algonquin Road
Arlington Heights, IL 60005
1-888-4PLASTIC
www.plasticsurgery.org
Has information on plastic surgery. Call for the names of qualified professionals in your area.

Association for the Protection of the Elderly (APE)

528A Columbia Avenue, Suite 127

Lexington, SC 29072

1–800–569–7345

fax: 1–803–356–6212

e–mail: ape@apeape.org

www.apeape.org

Has information about how to find a nursing home.

Cable News Network, Inc. (CNN)

www.cnn.com/HEALTH

Information about a variety of health issues.

Cancer Information Service (CIS)

1–800–4CANCER

www.cis.nci.nih.gov

Has answers to questions about cancer–related issues.

CBS Healthwatch

www.healthwatch.medscape.com

Has information on cancer and health issues.

Centers for Disease Control and Prevention (CDC)

1600 Clifton Road

Atlanta, GA 30333

National AIDS hotline: 1–800–342–2437

1–800–311–3435 *or* 1–404–639–3534

www.cdc.gov

Has information about various health care issues.

Combined Health Information Database

www.chid.nih.gov

Bibliographic database of various health care issues.

ConsumerLab.com

www.consumerlab.com

Provides consumers with results of independent tests of products affecting health.

Consumers Union of the U.S.

101 Truman Avenue

Yonkers, NY 10703-1057

1-914-378-2000

www.consumersunion.org

A nonprofit, independent organization that researches and tests consumer goods and services. Provides unbiased advice about products and services, health and nutrition, and other consumer concerns. Publishes *Consumer Reports* magazine, among other publications.

Council of Better Business Bureaus (CBBB)

4200 Wilson Boulevard, Suite 800

Arlington, VA 22203

1-703-276-0100

www.bbb.org

The CBBB is supported by local Better Business Bureaus (BBB). It serves as a spokesperson for business in the consumer field, supports consumer education programs, and works to arbitrate consumer complaints. Contact your local BBB for information specific to your area.

Federal Bureau of Investigation (FBI)

Health Care Fraud Unit

935 Pennsylvania Avenue NW, Room 7373

Washington, D.C. 20535

1-202-324-3000

fax: 1-202-324-8577

www.fbi.gov

The mission of the FBI's Health Care Fraud Unit is to investigate medical scams in multiple states and assist other law enforcement agencies with their health care fraud investigations.

Federal Trade Commission (FTC)

Health Care Fraud Bureau of Consumer Protection

CRC-240

Washington, D.C. 20580

1-877-FTC-HELP

www.ftc.gov

To report consumer fraud and misleading advertising.

Federation of State Medical Boards of the U.S.

400 Fuller Wiser Road, Suite 300

Euless, TX 76039-3857

1-817-868-4000

Ask about your physician's license and background.

Food and Drug Administration (FDA)

HFE-88

5600 Fisher's Lane

Rockville, MD 20857

Consumer hotline: 1-800-532-4440

Information on diet supplements: 1-800-FDA-1088

www.fda.gov

Has answers to questions about medicines, medical devices, and food supplements that are misrepresented, mislabeled, or harmful. Publishes *FDA Consumer* magazine. Access to MedWatch, the FDA Medical Products Reporting Program, whose purpose is to enhance the effectiveness of postmarketing surveillance of medical products as they are used in clinical practices and to rapidly identify significant health hazards associated with these products. Consumers can report an adverse event or illness related to a dietary supplement or a drug.

Fox News

www.foxnews.com/health/index.sml

News and information about health-related issues.

Georgia Council Against Health Care Fraud's Healthcare Reality Check

www.hcrc.org

Information about health and nutrition.

Health Care Financial Administration's (HCFA) Nursing Home Search

1 800 633 4227

OIG Hotline (to report Medicare fraud) 1-800-HHS-TIPS

www.medicare.gov

Users can search by zip code or state to see if a particular nursing home has been cited for problems. (If a nursing home is not listed, this does not mean it passed all inspections.) Provides a national directory of every Medicare- and Medicaid-certified facility. Has information on selecting a nursing home, Medicare violations.

Healthcare Reality Check

(See **Georgia Council Against Health Fraud's Healthcare Reality Check**)

Healthfinder

(See **U.S. Department of Health and Human Services**)

Healthgrades.com

www.healthgrades.com

Private company ratings of nursing homes; profiles on dentists, hospitals, fertility clinics, acupuncturists, naturopaths, physicians, chiropractors, mammography facilities, and hospitals.

Healthscout

www.healthscout.com

A news service that provides up to twenty health-related stories a day. A user can submit health interests and receive personalized newsletters and safety alerts by e-mail. Also has a section where health Web sites are rated.

International Bibliographic Information on Dietary Supplements (IBIDS database)

(See **Office of Dietary Supplements**)

Journal of the American Medical Association
(See **American Medical Association**)

Mayo Clinic Health Oasis
www.mayohealth.org
>Offers up-to-date information on health issues.

Medicaid
www.hcfa.gov/Medicaid
>Information on Medicaid benefits and health plans.

Medical Board of California
Division of Administration
1426 Howe Avenue, Suite 54
Sacramento, CA 95825-3236
www.medbd.ca.gov
1-916-263-2466 (general information)
1-916-263-2382 (to verify physician license and consumer information about doctors)
1-800-633-2322 (complaint line)
>Publishes a booklet with information about how to choose a doctor; has information about AIDS and cancer treatments.

Medical Matrix
www.medmatrix.org
>Directory of selected medical sites.

Medicare
1-800-Medicare
www.medicare.gov
>Information about health plans, nursing homes, and Medicare.

MEDLINEplus
(See **National Library of Medicine**)

Medscape
1-212-760-3100

www.medscape.com

Consumer news and articles about health issues; drug database with information on more than 200,000 drug products; access to NLM's MEDLINE and AIDSLine.

Michigan Consumer Guide to Nursing Homes
(Healthcare Association of Michigan)

www.hcam.org

Detailed checklist of what to look for and ask when checking into a long-term care facility.

Museum of Questionable Medical Devices

Bob McCoy, proprietor

201 Main Street SE

Minneapolis, MN

1-612-379-4046

www.mtn.org/quack

The world's largest display of questionable medical devices.

National Arthritis, Musculoskeletal and Skin Diseases Information

Box AMS

9000 Rockville Pike

Bethesda, MD 20892

1-301-495-4484

Answers questions about products and issues related to arthritis.

National Association of Consumer Agency Administrators (NACAA)

1010 Vermont Avenue NW, Suite 514

Washington, D.C. 20005

1-202-347-7395

fax: 1-202-347-2563

e-mail: nacaa@erols.com

www.nacaanet.org

Organization of federal, state, county, and local governmental consumer-protection agencies. The NACAA works to enhance consumer services, conducts seminars and public policy forums to promote consumer issues, and publishes a newsletter on scams and the latest enforcement activities.

National Cancer Institute
Public Inquiries Office
Building 31, Room 10A03
31 Center Drive, MSC 2580
Bethesda, MD 20892-2580
1-800-4CANCER *or* 1-301-435-3848
www.nci.nih.gov
   Provides information on issues related to cancer.

National Center for Complementary and Alternative Medicine (NCCAM)
P.O. Box 8218
Silver Spring, MD 20907-8218
1-888-644-6226
fax: 1-301-495-4957
www.nccam.nih.gov/nccam
   Conducts and supports research and training and disseminates information on complementary and alternative medicine to practitioners and the public.

National Center on Elder Abuse (NCEA)
1225 I Street NW, Suite 725
Washington, D.C. 20005
1-202-898-2586
fax: 1-202-898-2583
e-mail: NCEA@nasua.org
www.gwjapan.com/NCEA
   Provides information on elder abuse.

National Citizens' Coalition for Nursing Home Reform
1424 16th Street. NW, Suite 202
Washington, D.C. 20036-2211
1-202-332-2275

fax: 1–202–332–2949

www.nccnhr.org

Provides information on federal and state regulations, legislative policy development, and models and strategies to improve nursing home care.

National Consumers League (NCL)

1701 K Street NW, Suite 1201

Washington, D.C. 20006

1–202–835–3323 *or* 1–800–876–7060

fax: 1–202–835–0747

www.nclnet.org

The NCL is a nonprofit membership organization working for consumer health and safety protection and fairness in the marketplace and workplace.

National Council Against Health Fraud

(See **National Council for Reliable Health Information**)

National Council for Reliable Health Information (NCRHI)

Main office: William Jarvis, Ph.D., Executive Director

P.O. Box 1276

Loma Linda, CA 92354

1–909–824–4690

fax: 1–909–824–4838

A private, nonprofit, voluntary health agency focusing on health misinformation, fraud and quackery as public health problems. Lists reliable and unreliable health-related Web sites.

National Fraud Information Center of the National Consumers League

P.O. Box 65868

Washington, D.C. 20035

1–800–876–7060

www.fraud.org

Nonprofit consumer agency fighting telemarketing fraud.

National Institute on Aging (NIA)

P.O. Box 8057

Gaithersburg, MD 20898-8057

1-800-222-2225

www.nih.gov/nia

Provides information on health and aging.

National Library of Medicine (NLM)

8600 Rockville Pike

Bethesda, MD 20894

1-888-FIND-NLM *or* 1-301-594-5983

e-mail: custserv@nlm.nih.gov

www.nlm.nih.gov

Includes: MEDLINE, references from biomedical journals; MEDLINE-plus, answers to health questions; ClinicalTrials.gov, information about clinical research studies; and DIRLINE, a directory of health organizations.

National Library of Medicine, Specialized Information Services

HIV/AIDS resources: 1-301-496-3147 *or* 1-301-496-1131

fax: 1-301-480-3537

e-mail: aids@aids.nlm.nih.gov

www.sis.nlm.nih.gov/hotlines

Listing of toll-free phone numbers that provide information on AIDS, cancer, maternal and child health, aging, substance abuse, disabilities, and mental health.

National Patient Safety Foundation (at the AMA)

515 North State Street, 8th Floor

Chicago, IL 60610

1-312-464-4848

fax: 1-312-464-4154

e-mail: npsf@ama-assn.org

www.ama-assn.org

The NPSF's mission is to improve patient safety in the delivery of health care. Provides links to a variety of Web sites with information relative to its mission.

National Practitioner Data Bank and Healthcare Integrity and Protection Data Bank

P.O. Box 10832

Chantilly, VA 20153-0832

1-800-767-6732

www.npdb.com

A central source on physicians, dentists, and health care workers practicing in the U.S. Only available to those in the medical community, not the general public.

National Women's Health Information Center (NWHIC)

1-800-994-WOMAN

e-mail: 4woman@soza.com

www.4woman.gov

A U.S. Public Health Service Web site that links to over 1,000 other women's-health Web sites, including federal, government-screened private organizations, and more than 2,700 federal documents on women's health.

NBC

www.msnbc.com/news/HEALTH_front.asp

News and information about health-related issues.

New England Journal of Medicine

10 Shattuck Street

Boston, MA 02115 6094

1-617-734-9800

fax: 1 617 739-9864

www.nejm.org/content/index.asp

Medical journal that contains information on various health issues.

Nursing Home Abuse and Neglect Information Center
1-510-235-5021 *or* 1-408-997-9540
fax: 1-510-232-2570
e-mail: dlrasor@quitam.com
www.nursinghomeabuse.com/index/html.

Privately operated site that has information on nursing-home abuse—what to look for and what can be done about it.

Office of Dietary Supplements (ODS)
Building 31, Room 1B25
31 Center Drive, MSC 2086
Bethesda, MD 20892-2096
1-301-435-2920
fax: 1-301-480-1845
e-mail: ods@nih.gov
www.odp.od.nih.gov/ods

The ODS supports research and disseminates research results in the area of dietary supplements. The International Bibliographic Information on Dietary Supplements (IBIDS) can be accessed from their Web site. IBIDS is a database of facts about dietary supplements that searches existing medical, botanical, agricultural, chemical, and pharmaceutical databases. It also offers links to other scientific, government, and professional sites related to dietary supplements.

Public Citizen
Health Research Group
1600 20th St. NW
Washington, D.C. 20009
1-202-588-1000
www.citizen.org

Founded by Ralph Nader in 1971, Public Citizen is a nonprofit consumer advocacy organization. It publishes a consumer guide of doctors who've been sanctioned by state medical boards.

Quackwatch

www.quackwatch.com

Dr. Stephen Barrett's Web site, with information on medical quackery and health fraud. Other projects of Quackwatch include: NutriWatch (www.nutriwatch.org) operated by Stephen Barrett, M.D., and Manfred Kroger Ph.D.; and MLM Watch (www.mlmwatch.org) operated by Stephen Barrett, M.D.

SearchPointe

www.searchpointe.com

This site's Doctor Search provides information on licensed medical doctors and doctors of osteopathy in the U.S. The Chiropractor Search informs consumers about doctors of chiropractic with active licenses.

U.S. Department of Health and Human Services

Headquarters

Hubert H. Humphrey Building

200 Independence Avenue SW

Washington, D.C. 20201

www.hhs.gov

Has links to its operating divisions including NIH, FDA, CDC, HCFA, and AoA. A portal to Web sites of multi-agency health initiatives and activities of the U.S. Department of Health and Human Services and other federal departments including the Office of the Surgeon General, the Office of Public Health and Science, and the Office of Disease Prevention and Health Promotion. Contains information about dietary guidelines.

www.hrsa.dhhs.gov or www.healthfinder.gov

Free guide to reliable health information including information about alternative medicine, Medicare, choosing quality care, government health news, medical dictionaries, databases, and more.

U.S. Postal Inspection Service

www.usps.com/postalinspectors

Investigates mail fraud. Report mail fraud online.

U.S. Postal Service

Chief Postal Inspector

475 L'Enfant Plaza SW

Washington, D.C. 20260-2100

1-202-268-4267

www.new.usps.gov

Information about mail fraud. Report mail fraud to your local postal inspector.

Specific addresses for the following may be found in the City, County, and State Government listings in the white pages of your telephone directory:

District Attorney's Office

State Attorney General's Office

Both the District Attorney's Office and the State Attorney General's Office investigate and prosecute fraud cases.

State or Local Health Department

State or local Poison Control

Home and Community Services

Social and Health Services

These are sources of information for a variety of health issues. They are known by a variety of names depending on locality.

State Board of Medical Examiners

State Office on Aging

The state medical board is responsible for licensing doctors. Their powers include the ability to revoke and suspend medical licenses. The Office on Aging often contains the Office of the State Long-Term Care Ombudsman where you can locate the local ombudsman for your area.

Selected Bibliography

"$120.5M Aetna Verdict Upheld." *Associated Press Online* (29 March 1999).

Acu-Stop brochure. © 1992 Acu-Stop.

Alexander, Brian. "Health Tonic Hazard: Colloidal Minerals Are Flying off the Shelves of Health Food Stores—and Could Be Dangerous." *Self* (March 1997): 62.

AMA Council on Mental Health. "The Sick Physician: Impairment by Psychiatric Disorders, Including Alcoholism and Drug Dependence." *JAMA* 223 (1973): 684–87.

American Herbal Products Association. "FDA Issues Final Rule for Structure/Function Statements." *AHPA: News, Events, and Announcements* (7 January 2000). www.ahpa.org/fda.html.

Armstrong, David, and Elizabeth Metzger Armstrong. *The Great American Medicine Show*. New York: Prentice-Hall, 1991.

Aronovitz, Leslie G. "Medicaid, Federal and State Leadership Needed to Control Fraud and Abuse." *U.S. General Accounting Office/Health, Education and Human Services Division*, Pub. 00-30.

Baldwin, DeWitt C. Jr., et al. "Substance Use Among Senior Medical Students: A Survey of 23 Medical Schools." *JAMA* 265, no. 16 (24 April 1991): 2074–78.

Barrett, Stephen. "Commercial Hair Analysis: A Cardinal Sign of Quackery." *Quackwatch*. www.quackwatch.com/01QuackeryRelatedTopics/hair.html.

———. "Electrodiagnostic Devices." *Quackwatch*. www.quackwatch.com/01QuackeryRelatedTopics/electro.html.

———. "Gastrointestinal Quackery: Colonics, Laxatives and More." *Quackwatch*. www.quackwatch.com.

———. "Index to "Fad" Diagnoses." *Quackwatch*. www.quackwatch.com.

Barrett, Stephen, M.D., and William T. Jarvis, Ph.D. "'Holistic Dentistry': A Brief Overview." *Quackwatch*. www.quackwatch.com/01QuackeryRelatedTopics/holisticdent.html.

Barrett, Stephen, M.D., and William T. Jarvis, Ph.D., eds. *The Health Robbers: A Close Look at Quackery in America*. Buffalo, N.Y.: Prometheus Books, 1993.

Beecher, H. K. "The Powerful Placebo." *JAMA* 159 (1955): 1602–6.

Biegelman, Martin T. *Protecting with Distinction: A Postal Inspection Service History of the Mail Fraud Statute*. U.S. Postal Inspection Service, 1999.

Blankenheim, Tracy A. "Problem Homes to Face Immediate Penalties, Fines." *McKnight's Long-Term Care News* 21, no. 1 (14 January 2000): 17.

———. "Report Calls 13 Percent of Therapy 'Not Medically Necessary.'" *McKnight's Long-Term Care News* 20, no. 14 (6 October 1999): 22.

Bowers, Mark. "AIDS Fraud Article." *AIDS Health Fraud Task Force of California* (March 1996). www.aidsfraud.com/Articles/AIDS_Fraud_Article/aids_fraud_article.html.

Bragg, Rick. "Quest for Beauty Went Awry at Hands of a Fake Surgeon, Miami Police Say." *New York Times* 149, no. 51668 (7 October 1999): A16.

Brecher, Edward M., and the Editors of *Consumer Reports*. "The Consumers Union Report on Licit and Illicit Drugs." (1972). www.ukcia.org/lib/cunion/cu8.htm.

British Columbia Cancer Agency. "Psychic Surgery." www.bccancer.bc.ca.

Brown, John Ronald. Statement regarding perceived slander committed on *Inside Edition* television program (14 June 1989).

Budiansky, Stephen. "New Snake Oil, Old Pitch." *U.S. News and World Report* 101, no. 23 (8 December 1986).

Burrow, James G. *AMA: Voice of American Medicine*. Baltimore: The Johns Hopkins Press, 1963.

Carroll, Robert T. "Crystal Power." *The Skeptics Dictionary*. (1998) www.skepdic.com/crystals.html.

Carson, Gerald. *One for a Man, Two for a Horse*. Garden City, N.Y.: Doubleday and Co., Inc., 1961.

Ciotti, Paul. "Why Did He Cut off That Man's Leg?" *LA Weekly* 22, no. 4 (17 December 1999): 24–33.

Cohen, Elizabeth. "Dieters Rah-Rah Over Fen-Phen." *CNN.com* (17 December 1996). www.cnn.com/HEALTH/9612/17/fen.phen.

Coleman, Ellen. "Herbal Crystallization Analysis." *Healthcare Reality Check*. www.hcrc.org/faqs/herbcrys.html.

"Companies Recall Herbs That Contain Diabetes Drug." *Associated Press* (23 March 2000). www.cnn.com/2000/HEALTH/alternative/03/23/herb.recall.ap/index/html.

Cooper, Anderson, and Carole Simpson. "Battle Lines Drawn Among Patients and Healthcare." *ABC World News Sunday* (24 May 1998).

"Crystal Physics Technology." Advertisement for the BioElectric Shield. www.lifeenrichment.com/yogamain/bioyoga.htm.

Dardik, I. I. "The Origin of Disease and Health Heart Waves." *Cycles* 46, no. 3 (1996).

Davis, Robert. "Liposuction Death Rate 'Unacceptable.'" *USA Today* (18 January 2000). www.usatoday.com/life/health/plastic/lhpla002.htm.

"Dentist Agrees to Settle Medicaid Fraud Case." Texas Health and Human Services Commission. www.hhsc.state.tx.us/news/release/dentist.htm.

Derbyshire, Robert C., M.D. "The Make-Believe Doctors." In *The Health Robbers*, edited by Stephen Barrett, M.D., and William T. Jarvis, Ph.D. Buffalo, N.Y.: Prometheus Books, 1993.

"Dietary Supplements Worrisome Contaminants Found." *Mayo Clinic Health Oasis* (31 August 1998). www.mayohealth.org/mayo/9808/htm/diet.htm.

Doyle, Paul J. (Administrative Trial Judge). Letter to the Board of Medical Quality Assurance, State of California. (22 November 1977).

Dryer, L. M. L. "Bottled Water: A Critical Look." *Healthcare Reality Check*. www.hcrc.org/contrib/dryer/bottled.html.

Ecenbarger, William. "How Honest Are Dentists?" *Reader's Digest* 150, no. 898 (February 1997): 50–56.

Eichenwald, Kurt, and Gina Kolata. "A Doctor's Drug Studies Turn into Fraud." *New York Times* (16 May 1999).

———. Drug Trials Hide Conflicts for Doctors. *New York Times* (17 May 1999).

Eisenberg, Carol. "HMOs Face a Backlash: Consumers Fuel Fight for 'Patient Rights.'" *Newsday* 6 (7 June 1998): A05.

Ernst, E. "Colonic Irrigation and the Theory of Autointoxication: A Triumph of Ignorance over Science." *J Clin Gastroenter* 24 (1997): 196–98.

Farley, Dixie. "Dietary Supplements: Making Sure Hype Doesn't Overwhelm Science." *Food and Drug Administration* (November 1993). www.fda.gov/bbs/topics/CONSUMER/CON00259.html.

"FDA Panel Says Single Saline Implant Safe—With Warnings." Eileen O'Connor and the Associated Press, contributors *CNN.com* (2 March 2000). www.cnn.com/2000/HEALTH/03/03/breast.implants/index.html.

Federal Trade Commission. "Bogus Business Opportunity Sellers Settle FTC Charges; Consumers and Franchises Victims of Phony Alcohol 'Neutralizer.'" Press release (28 May 1997). www.ftc.gov/opa/1997/9705/boci.htm.

———. "Decision and Order in the Matter of New Vision International, Inc., et al." FTC Docket No. C-3856. (Issued 3 March 1999).

———. "Dietary Supplements: An Advertising Guide for Industry." *Federal Trade Commission.* www.ftc.gov/bcp/conline/pubs/buspubs/dietsupp.htm.

———. "'Hair Farmer' Settles FTC Charges." Press release (12 November 1998). www.ftc.gov/opa/1998/9811/sabal1.htm.

———. "Infomercial Marketers Settle FTC Charges." Press release (13 January 1998). www.ftc.gov/opa/1998/9801/megasyst.htm.

———. "Infomercials." *Federal Trade Commission.* www.ftc.gov/bcp/conline/pubs/products/info.htm.

———. "Marketers of 'The Enforma System' Settle FTC Charges of Deceptive Advertising for Their Weight Loss Products." Press release (26 April 2000). www.ftc.gov/opa/2000/04/index.htm.

———. "Marketers of 'Vitamin O' Settle FTC Charges of Making False Health Claims; Will Pay $375,000 for Consumer Redress." (1 May 2000). www.ftc.gov/opa.

———. "Medical Association Settles False Advertising Charges Over Promotion of 'Chelation Therapy.'" *Quackwatch.* www.quackwatch.com/02ConsumerProtection/ftcchelation.html.

————. "Multi-Level Marketing Company to Settle FTC Charges That It Made Unsubstantiated Claims That Its 'God's Recipe' Dietary Regimen Could Cure ADD/ADHD." (8 December 1998). www.ftc.gov/opa/1998/9812/nvi2.htm.

————. "Nu Skin to Pay $1.5 Million Penalty to Resolve FTC Charges over Fat-loss Claims for Supplements." (6 August 1997). www.ftc.gov.

————. "Operation Cure.all Cases." (1999). www.ftc.gov/opa/1999/9906/opcureall.htm (press release-proposed consents), www.ftc.gov/opa/1999/9909/fyi990920.htm (press release-final consent).

"Fen-Phen Maker Settles Suits for $3.75B." *USA Today* (7 October 1999). www.usatoday.com/life/health/diet/lhdie065.htm.

Ferrari, Susan. "Narrative statement by John Ronald Brown, memorandum." State of California Department of Consumer Affairs. (12 January 1983).

Fienberg, S. E., and D. H. Kaye. "Legal and Statistical Aspects of Some Mysterious Clusters." *Journal of the Royal Statistical Society,* series A, 154 (1991): 61–74. www.law.asu.edu/kaye/pubs/evid/clusters91JRSS.htm.

Food and Drug Administration. "Answers 09/15/1988: Homeopathy and 'Homeopathy.'" (15 September 1998). www.fda.gov/bbs/topics/ANSWERS/ANS00213.html.

————. "FDA/CFSAN Office of Special Nutritionals: Overview of Dietary Supplements." *FDA Center for Food Safety and Applied Nutrition* (May 1997, Updated April 1999). vm.cfsan.fda.gov/~dms.

————. "FDA Finalizes Rules for Claims on Dietary Supplements." *FDA Talk Paper* (5 January 2000). vm.cfsan.fda.gov/~lrd.

————. "FDA Warns Against Consuming Triax Metabolic Accelerator." *FDA Talk Paper* (11 November 1999). www.fda.gov/bbs/topics/ANSWERS/ANS00984.html.

————. "FDA Warns Against Drug Promotion of 'Herbal Fen-Phen.'"
FDA Talk Paper (6 November 1997).
vm.cfsan.fda.gov/~lrd/tpfenphn.html.

"Gas Grill Igniters: The Stimulator and Crystaldyne Pain Reliever."
Museum of Questionable Medical Devices.
www.mtn.org/quack/devices/stimul.htm.

Goodrum, Charles, and Helen Dalyrumple. *Advertising in America: The
First 200 Years.* New York: Harry N. Abrams, Inc., 1990.

Gorman, Christine. "Managed Care: Playing the HMO Game." *Time*
152, no. 2 (13 July 1998). www.pathfinder.com/time/magazine/
1998/dom/980713/cover1.html.

Gorski, Timothy. "Archives of Xenomedicine: Medical Myths and
Misperceptions." *Tarrant County Physician* 10 (1999).
www.hcrc.org/contrib/gorski/tcp99-10.html.

Green, Saul. "Chelation Therapy: Unproven Claims and Unsound
Theories." *Quackwatch.*
www.quackwatch.com/01QuackeryRelatedTopics/chelation.html.

Grimes, Kevin D., and Spencer M. Reese. "FTC Complaint for
Permanent Injunction Against Rose Creek Health Products."
(1999) *Grimes & Reese, P.L.L.C.*
www.directsaleslaw.com/library/cases/salesmark/rosecreekcmp.htm.

Gugliotta, Guy. "Health Concerns Grow Over Herbal Aids." *Washington
Post* (19 March 2000). www.washingtonpost.com/wp-dyn/articles/
A32685-2000Mar17.html.

Hansing, Linda M. "Don't Let Coding Errors Torpedo Your Managed
Care Contracts." *Medical Economics* 73, no. 18 (1996): 145–52.

"Hard Data." *McKnight's Long-Term Care News* 20, no. 10 (13 July 1999): 6.

"Health Hazards & Hoaxes." From the files of Ben Wilson, M.D. (1986).

Hellmich, N. "Pitching Pills That Lighten Wallets." *USA Today* (16
August 1999). www.usatoday.com/life/health/diet/lhdie051.htm.

"Herb–Drug Interactions: Natural Not Always Safe." *Mayo Clinic Health Oasis* (6 March 2000). www.mayohealth.org/mayo/0003/htm/herbdrug.htm.

Heymsfield, Steven B., et al. "*Garcinia cambogia* (Hydroxycitric Acid) as a Potential Antiobesity Agent." *JAMA* 280, no. 18 (11 November 1998): 1596–600.

Hiaasen, Carl. "Dr. Who? Get the Lowdown Before the Lift." *Miami Herald* (10 October 1999). www.herald.com.

Hilzenrath, David S. "At Stake in Senate Debate: HMOs' Shield Against Damage Suits." *Washington Post* (11 July 1999): A12.

Hwang, Mi Young. "Alternative Choices: What It Means to Use Nonconventional Medical Therapy." In *AMA Health Insight: Alternative Medicine,* edited by Richard M. Glass, M.D. www.ama-assn.org/insight/spec_con/patient/pat027.htm.

"Infomercial Marketers Settle FTC Charges." *CNN.com* (13 January 1998). www.cnn.com/CNN/bureaus/chicago/stories/9801/infomercial/index.htm.

Isaacs, L. C., and F. Bronner. Letter from the Department of Health & Human Services (29 August 1995).

Japan Ministry of Health and Welfare. "Okinawa Census Data." www.okinawa-ric.or.jp/virtualtown/movee/english/kiso01_e.htm.

Jarvis, William T., Ph.D. Dubious Dentistry: A Dental Continuing Education Course (course materials). School of Dentistry, Loma Linda University, 1990.

Jost, Kenneth. "Managed-Care Plans Are Drawing Criticism." *St. Louis Post-Dispatch Congressional Quarterly* (17 January 1998): A4.

Kaufman, Martin. *Homeopathy in America: The Rise and Fall of a Medical History.* Baltimore: The Johns Hopkins University Press, 1971.

Keung, Wing-Ming, and Bert Vallee. "Daidzin: A Potent, Selective Inhibitor of Human Mitochondrial Aldehyde Dehydrogenase." *Proc. Natl. Acad. Sci. USA* 90 (1993): 1247–51.

Kurtzweil, Paula. "A 'Washed-Up' Snake Oil Scheme." *FDA Consumer* 30, no. 7 (September 1996): 30.

———. "An FDA Guide to Dietary Supplements." *FDA Consumer* (September October 1998; Revised January 1999), Publication no. (FDA) 99-2323. www.vm.cfsan.fda.gov/~dms/.

———. "Internet Sales of Bogus HIV Test Kits Result in First-of-Kind Wire Fraud Conviction." *FDA Consumer* 33, no. 4 (July–August 1999): 34–35.

———. "Ozone Generators Generate Prison Terms for Couple (Investigator's Reports)." *FDA Consumer* 33, no. 6 (November–December 1999): 36–37.

Larkin, Marilynn. "Internet Accelerates Spread of Bogus Cancer Cure." *The Lancet* 353, no. 9149 (23 January 1999): 331.

le Bissell, C., P. Haberman, and R. L. Williams. "Pharmacists Recovering from Alcohol and Other Drug Addictions: An Interview Study." *American Pharmacy* NS29 (1989): 391–402.

Lemonick, Michael D. "The Dark Side of Diet Pills (Restrictions on Redux and Fen-Phen)." *Time* 150, no. 12 (22 September 1997): 81(1). www.pathfinder.com/time/magazine/1997/dom/970922/health.dark_side_of_.html.

Lewis, Carol. "Phony Doc Sentenced to Real Jail Time." *FDA Consumer* 33, no. 1 (January–February 1999): 35–36.

Lumpkin, Murray M., M.D. "FDA Public Health Advisory on Dietary Supplement." *Center for Food Safety and Applied Nutrition* (10 February 2000).www.americanutra.com/press.html.

MacFarlane, Ellen B. *Legwork: An Inspiring Journey Through a Chronic Illness.* New York: USA Drew Books, 1994.

"Maker of Weight-Loss Pill Forced to Pay $8 Million." *USA Today* (20 July 1999). www.usatoday.com/life/health.diet/lhdie044.htm.

"Malpractice Judgment Against Hal Huggins." *National Council Against Health Fraud Newsletter* 19, no. 1 (January–February 1996): 2(2).

Marchant, G. "No Anesthetic, No Knife; Bail-Jumping Reverend Antonia Agpaoa Will Heal You with His Bare Hands." *Vancouver Magazine* 7 (1978): 45–47.

Mayorkas, Alejandro N., U.S. Attorney, Central District of CA. "Beverly Hills Doctor Accused in Massive Medicare Fraud Case." Press release (13 January 1998). www.usdoj.gov/usao/cac/pr/1998/98-09.htm.

McBride, Judy. "Antioxidant Power of Natural Product Supplements Highly Variable." Agricultural Research Service, USDA, *ARS News Service* (9 August 1999). www.americanutra.com/press.html.

McClellan, Gerald. Senior Special Investigator, State of California Dept. of Consumer Affairs, to Ronald L. Kramer, California Board of Medical Quality Assurance (20 December 1989): 1–3.

———. Senior Investigator, Medical Board of California, to Stacy L. Running, Deputy District Attorney (21 July 1998): 1–2.

———. Senior Investigator, Medical Board of California, Division of Medical Quality to Stacy L. Running (2 September 1998). Re: John Ronald Brown.

McIntyre, B. W., and M. W. Hamolsky. "The Impaired Physician and the Role of the Board of Medical Licensure and Discipline." *Rhode Island Medicine* 81 (1994): 101–5.

McKenzie, John. "Disciplining Incompetent Doctors." *ABC World News Tonight.* (11 January 2000). www.abcnews.go.com/onair/WorldNews Tonight/wnt_000111_CL_BadDrs_feature.html.

"Medicaid Fraud Report." State of Nevada, Office of the Attorney General (May 1998). www.state.nv.us/ag/mfcu/naag.htm.

Medical Board of California. "Status report on medical license of Carl J. Reich." www.healthwatcher.net/Quackerywatch/Coral-Calcium/reich-california-license.html.

Merkle, G.E., et al., eds. *Politics, Science and Cancer: The Laetrile Phenomenon.* Boulder, CO: Westview Press, 1980.

Millikan, Larry E. "Alcoholism Among Health Professionals: Prevalence and Special Problems." *Clinics in Dermatology* 17 (1999): 361–63.

Mitka, Mike "Unacceptable Nursing Home Deaths Unautopsied." *JAMA* 280, no. 12 (23 September 1998): 1038(1).

Morris, Jim. "Loosening Controls on Medicaid Fraud." *Houston Chronicle* (1 October 1995). www.chron.com.

"Muscle Building: Do Andro, Creatine Work?" *Mayo Clinic Health Oasis* (9 November 1998). www.mayohealth.org/mayo/9811/htm/muscle.htm.

Museum of Questionable Medical Devices. "Albert Abrams, A.M., M.D., LL.D., F.R.M.S." *Great American Quacks.* www.mtn.org/quack/amquacks/abrams.htm.

National Cancer Institute. "NCI Fact Sheet: Paclitaxel (Taxol) and Related Anticancer Drugs." www.oncolink.upenn.edu/pdq_html/6/engl/600715.html.

National Council Against Health Care Fraud (now known as the National Council for Reliable Health Information). "NCAHF Position Paper on Homeopathy." Loma Linda, California, 1994. www.ncahf.org/pp/homeop.html.

Nordenberg, Tamar. "The Death of the Party." *FDA Consumer* 34, no. 2 (2 March 2000): 14.

"Nursing Facility Measure: Ancillary Costs Per Resident Day." *McKnight's Long-Term Care News* 20, no. 3 (15 September 1999): 10.

"Oregon Doctor Fined over Internet Prescriptions." Reuters Limited (31 March 2000). On America Online.

Parrish, M. "How Did This Man Convince Everyone He Was a Doctor?" *Medical Economics* 23 (September 1996): 89–97.

Patrick, William. *The Food and Drug Administration (Know Your Government)*. New York: Chelsea House Publishers, 1988.

Pfingst, Paul J., and Stacy L. Running. Trial brief (21 September 1999). *The People of the State of California v. John Ronald Brown.*

Polevoy, Terry. "Smart Chicks of Okinawa—a Tale of Broken Yolks, Empty Promises and Health Robbery." www.healthwatcher.net/ Quackerywatch/Coral-Calcium/coral_calcium.html.

Pontolillo, James. "Colloidal Mineral Supplements: Unnecessary and Potentially Hazardous." *Quackwatch.* www.quackwatch.com/ 01QuackeryRelatedTopics/DSH/colloidalminerals.html.

"The Problem with Fen-Phen." www.loop.com/~bkrentzman/meds/ Phen-Fen/phen.serotonin.html.

"The Radio Disease Killer: ERA Quack Diagnostic Instrument." *American Artifacts*, no. 39. www.americanartifacts.com/smma/abrams/rdk.htm.

Raines, K. "Dr. Albert Abrams and the E.R.A." www.premier1.net/~raines/abrams.html.

Randi, James (Host). "The World's Greatest Scams." Aired on the History Channel (1 April 2000).

Roberts, A. H., et al. "The Power of Nonspecific Effects in Healing: Implications for Psychological and Biological Treatments." *Clin Psychol Rev* 13 (1993): 375–91.

Root-Bernstein, Robert, and Michele Root-Bernstein. *Honey, Mud, Maggots and Other Medical Marvels.* Boston: Houghton Mifflin, 1997.

Rosa, Linda, et al. "A Close Look at Therapeutic Touch." *JAMA* 279 no. 13 (1 April 1998): 1005-10.

Rowland, Rhonda. "Liposuction Blamed in Five Deaths." *CNN.com* (12 May 1999). www.cnn.com/HEALTH/9905/12/liposuction. deaths.02/index.html.

Scanlon, William J. "California Nursing Homes: Federal and State Oversight Inadequate to Protect Residents in Homes with Serious Care Violations." *U.S. General Accounting Office/Health, Education and Human Services Division,* Pub. 98-219: 1–16.

————. "Nursing Homes: Enhanced HCFA Oversight of State Programs Would Better Ensure Quality Care." *U.S. General Accounting Office/Health, Education and Human Services Division,* Pub. 00-27: 1.

————. "Nursing Homes: HCFA Initiatives to Improve Care Are Under Way but Will Require Continued Commitment." *U.S. General Accounting Office/Health, Education and Human Services Division,* Pub. 99–155.

Schulte, Fred. "Vanity Medicine. Hope, Hype, and Risk." *Sun-Sentinel (South Florida)* (11 December 1999). www.sun-sentinel.com.

Schulte, Fred, and Jenni Bergal. "Cosmetic Surgery: The Hidden Dangers." (series) *Sun-Sentinel (South Florida).* www.sun-sentinel.com.

————. "Lack of Licenses Did Not Stop Them from Performing Surgery." *Sun-Sentinel (South Florida)* (14 December 1999). www.sun-sentinel.com.

————. "Self-Proclaimed Surgeon Serving Time in Fraud Case." *Sun-Sentinel (South Florida)* (14 December 1999). www.sun-sentinel.com.

Schulte, James E. "An Impaired Doctor Cost His Colleagues $5 Million." *Medical Economics* 67, no. 11 (4 June 1990): 44–50.

————. *Fraud & Abuse Prevention: What Physicians Need to Know.* Texas Medical Association, 1998.

————. *Preventing Medical Malpractice Suits: A Handbook for Doctors and Those Who Work with Them.* Seattle: Hogrefe and Huber, 1995.

"Serotonin and Eating Disorders." *Medical Sciences Bulletin* 10 (1994). www.pharminfo.com/pubs/msb/seroton.html.

Shellow, R. A., and P. G. Coleman. "Fitness to Practice Medicine: A Question of Conduct, Not Mental Illness." *Journal of the Florida Medical Association* 8 (1994): 101–5.

Sherill, Robert. "A Year in Corporate Crime." *Nation* 264, no. 13 (7 April 1997): 11(8).

Shomon, Mary. "Synthroid Class Action Lawsuit Settlement Approved." www.thyroid.about.com.

———. "Synthroid Manufacturer Settles with 37 States." (29 July 1999). www.thyroid.about.com.

———. "Synthroid Under Siege." (2 February 1999). www.thyroid. about.com/health/thyroid/library/weekly/aa022899.htm.

Shryock, Richard Harrison. *Medicine and Society in America, 1660–1860.* New York: New York University Press, 1960.

Skolnick, Andrew A. "Surf's Up for Health Fraud Investigators" (Medical News & Perspectives). *JAMA* 278, no. 21 (3 December 1997): 1725.

Smith, J.W. *The World's Wasted Wealth 2: Save Our Wealth, Save Our Environment.* Cambria, CA: Institute for Economic Democracy, 1994. Excerpted at www.slonet.org/~ied/index.html.

Sobue, T., et al. "Lung Cancer Incidence Rates by Histologic Type in High- and Low-Risk Areas: A Population-Based Study in Osaka, Okinawa, and Saku-Nagano." *J Epidemiol* 9, no. 3 (June 1999): 134–42.

Spaeth, Dennis. "HHS Touts Decline in Medicare Overpayments." *ADA News* (10 February 1999). www.ada.org/adapco/daily/archives/9902/0210med.html.

St. Paul Fire & Marine Ins. Co. v. Mori, 486 N.W.2d 803 (Minn. App. 1992).

"Stabilized Oxygen." www.aabhealth.com/stabilized_oxygen.htm.

Stanley, Christina, M.D., Deputy Medical Examiner, San Diego County. "Autopsy on Philip Bondy, 25 August 1998."

"State Health Director Warns Consumers About Prescription Drugs in Herbal Products." Sacramento, CA. Press release. (15 February 2000). www.americanutra.com/press.html.

"State's Largest Dental Plan Posts Record Cost-Savings." BW HealthWire/CA-Delta-Dental (20 April 1999). www.businesswire.com.

Stewart, James B. *Blind Eye: How the Medical Establishment Let a Doctor Get Away with Murder.* New York: Simon & Schuster, 1999.

Stolberg, Sheryl Gay. "Trade Agency Finds Web Slippery with Snake Oil." *New York Times* 148, no. 51564 (25 June 1999): A16.

Stone, M. H., et al. "Effects of In-Season (5 Weeks) Creatine and Pyruvate Supplementation on Anaerobic Performance and Body Composition in American Football Players." *Int J Sport Nutr* 9 (1999): 146–65.

Stovall, Gary, and Steve Lindley "Officer's report concerning: 192(b) P.C. manslaughter. Victim: Bondy, Philip. Case no. 9803565. Accused: Brown, John Ronald, Date 05/11/98." (20 May 1999).

"Supplements Associated with Illnesses and Injuries." *FDA Consumer* (September–October 1998). Source: *FDA Statement Before Senate Committee on Labor and Human Resources* (21 October 1993). www.fda.gov/fdac/features/1998/dietchrt.html.

Sweet, Cheryl A. "Scents and Nonsense: Does Aromatherapy Stink?" *American Council on Science and Health.* www.acsh.org/publications/priorities/0904/aromatherapy.html.

"Taking Vitamin Supplements Is as American as Apple Pie." *Milwaukee Journal Sentinel* report published in "To Your Health" section of the *San Diego Union-Tribune* (20 March 2000): E-3.

"Theronoid Electromagnetic Solenoid." *American Artifacts.* www.americanartifacts.com/smma/thero.htm.

Thomas, M. Carroll. "Nine Babies Died Before This Doctor Was Stopped." *Medical Economics* 67, no. 19 (1 October 1990): 48–62.

Thompson, Mark. "Shining a Light on Abuse." *Time* 152, no. 5 (3 August 1998): 42(2).

Turner, Judith A. "Placebo Effects on Pain." *Healthline Magazine* 14, no. 4 (1995).

U.S. Postal Inspection Service. "Postal News: kNOw FRAUD Takes Aim at Illegal Telemarketers." *U.S. Postal Inspection Service* (17 November 1999). www.usps.gov/news/press/99/kNOw.htm.

————. "Postal News: Postal Service Takes Another Step to Prevent Mail Fraud." *U.S. Postal Inspection Service,* Release No. 21 (25 March 1999). www.usps.gov/news/press/99/99021new.htm.

United States Postal Service v. Aerobic Life Industries, Inc. and William Reeves, P.S. Docket No. FR 96-282 (17 July 1996).

United States Postal Service v. Dennis P. Wilkie dba Amazing Products, Inc. and Dennis P. Wilkie, Docket No. FR 99-122 (18 August 1999).

"UNITEDHEALTHCARE INTRODUCES CARE COORDINA-TION." (9 November 1999). www.unitedhealthgroup.com/press/pressreleases/991109ccoord.html.

"Use of Enemas Is Limited." *FDA Consumer* 18, no. 6 (1984): 33.

"Violating Standard of Care Basis for Patient's Award." *American Medical News* 11, no. 1 (9 November 1998).

Wallace, Robert. "An Arthritis 'Expert' Under Fire over Best-Selling Book." *Life* (25 March 1957).

Whitcomb, Dan. "California Jury Orders HMO to Pay $116 Million in Damages." *Reuters* (20 January 1999).

Whitlock, Charles R. *Chuck Whitlock's Scam School.* New York: Macmillan, 1997.

————. *Easy Money.* New York: Kensington Publishing Co., 1994.

Wilson, Benjamin, M.D. "The Rise and Fall of Laetrile." *Quackwatch.* www.quackwatch.com.

"Wisconsin Law Will Help Patients Fight HMO Decisions." *Oregonian* 150, no. 50, 152 (14 May 2000), first edition: A4.

"World's Worst Doctor." *Inside Edition.* (Aired 17 February 1989).

Young, James Harvey. *The Medical Messiahs: A Social History of Health Quackery in Twentieth-Century America*. Princeton, N.J.: Princeton University Press, 1967.

————. *The Toadstool Millionaires: A Social History of Patent Medicines in America Before Federal Regulation*. Princeton, N.J.: Princeton University Press, 1961.

Zarrella, John. "Patients Disfigured by Alleged Phony Physician Bring Suit." *CNN.com* (6 October 1999). www.cnn.com/US/9910/06/phony.physician/.

Zoglin, Richard. "It's Amazing! Call Now! Infomercials Are Filling the Late-Night Hours with Tacky Pitches for Everything from Kitchen Tools to Baldness Cures." *Time* 137, no. 24 (17 June 1991): 71.

About the Author

Following a successful career in business, Chuck Whitlock began his career in broadcasting when he came to the attention of Oprah Winfrey's producers as the author of *Easy Money*, his first book on white-collar crime. After the first of several appearances on *Oprah*, he began to produce and anchor a regular news segment broadcast for Portland Oregon's KGW and on the NBC News satellite feed.

As an independent producer for the 1995 *Inside Edition* segment "Medicare Sting," Chuck was a recipient of several awards for investigative reporting. In 1996, "Medicare Sting" won him the National Headliner Award for Outstanding Investigative Reporting. In 1995–96 he was contracted to produce over fifty segments of *Hard Copy* on scams, con artists, and consumer issues. The same year he also hosted a weekly radio show.

In 1997 he published *Scam School* (Macmillan) and joined *Extra* as an investigative correspondent.

Currently, Whitlock speaks to audiences across the United States about how to avoid being victimized. He has shared his knowledge and experiences on such television programs as *Oprah, Today, Regis and Kathie Lee, The Charles Grodin Show, The Maury Povich Show, Geraldo, Sally Jessy Raphael, The Jenny Jones Show, Home & Family*, and others, as well as numerous radio shows.